NUTRIPOINTS

Dr Roy E. Vartabedian

NUTRIPOINTS was developed by Dr
Roy E. Vartabedian of the Cooper Clinic
in Dallas, Texas. He is an enthusiastic
promoter of health through proper nutrition. His Nutripoints programme has
been successfully used for several years
at the world-renowned Cooper Clinic in
Dallas, Texas, where he is Executive
Director of the In-Residence and Com-
munity Wellness Programs. He holds a
Doctor of Health Science degree and a
Bachelor of Public Health in Nutrition.
He lectures widely on nutrition and
health.

Kathy Matthews

Kathy Matthews is a writer specializing
in health and nutrition. She is the co-
author of the bestselling *Medical
Makeover*, and collaborated with
Sophia Loren on *On Women and
Beauty* and with Christie Brinkley on
Complete Outdoor Fitness Book.

Dr Roy E. Vartabedian

and Kathy Matthews

NUTRIPOINTS

The Breakthrough
Nutritional Programme

GRAFTON BOOKS
A Division of the Collins Publishing Group

LONDON GLASGOW
TORONTO SYDNEY AUCKLAND

Grafton Books
A Division of the Collins Publishing Group
8 Grafton Street, London W1X 3LA

Published by Grafton Books 1990

Neither the Nutripoints concept nor this book is sponsored
or affiliated with Nutri/System Inc. or the Nutri/System®
Weight Loss Programme.

A CIP catalogue record for this book
is available from the British Library

ISBN 0-246-13567-0
    0-246-13702-9 (Pbk)

Printed in Great Britain by
William Collins Sons & Co. Ltd, Glasgow

ACKNOWLEDGEMENTS

I owe a debt of gratitude to Dr Kenneth Cooper for his assistance in making this book possible. Dr Cooper's application of a point system to exercise in his landmark book, *Aerobics*, inspired me to apply this simple, practical concept to nutrition. In addition, his support in allowing me to devote time and energy to this book while directing the In-Residence Programs at the Aerobics Center made the project possible. By introducing me to his agent, Herbert M. Katz, he made this book a reality.

I am also deeply indebted to Herbert Katz. In addition to undertaking the standard responsibilities as the agent for *Nutripoints*, Herb acted as the 'godfather' of the book from its inception, becoming its first champion and promoter as well as a thoughtful and discerning reader. His guidance throughout the publishing process has been invaluable.

Bill Shinker of Harper & Row has been a galvanizing force. His marketing vision and energetic commitment to *Nutripoints* have from the beginning made my association with his company an exciting experience.

Larry Ashmead, my editor at Harper & Row, has provided the enthusiasm that has kept *Nutripoints* on course right from the beginning. His immediate appreciation of the book's concept and his unflagging support have been greatly appreciated.

Margaret Wimberger, also of Harper & Row, has been a meticulous reader and has contributed to the ultimate cohesion of the book.

My thanks to Mike Smith and Suzan Lewis, founders of Constructive Solutions, for their hard work. All the mathematical formulations and computations for *Nutripoints* were completed efficiently and accurately through their efforts, contributing to the book's scientific validity.

Georgia Kostas, R.D., M.P.H., Director of Clinical Nutrition at the Cooper Clinic, provided major portions of our initial data base and assisted in additional USDA data.

Kathleen Duran, R.D., Assistant Director, In-Residence Programs, acted as my nutritional consultant.

Ava Bursau, M.S., Associate Director, In-Residence Programs, is my able associate who helped keep things running smoothly in the In-Residence Programs and allowed me to focus on the book.

Susan Hill, my data-processing specialist, performed the herculean task of plugging 50,000 pieces of information into the computer in order to analyse all the foods found in *Nutripoints*.

Linda Zeiner and Susan Wampler, my executive secretary, worked on the major project of alphabetizing the food lists.

Scott Dyer of Tom Thumb Food Stores allowed me to obtain information on brand name foods at his facilities in North Dallas.

I am grateful to all the manufacturers who sent information on their products, allowing us to make complete and accurate analyses of their ingredients.

TO MY GRANDMA,
LOUISE VARTABEDIAN

It was my Grandma Louise's energy, positive attitude, and zest for living, combined with her compelling interest in foods that were 'poisons' or 'wonder foods' that inspired me to undertake nutrition as my life's work. Grandma Louise lived well into her eighties. My wish is that you may benefit from the culmination of my grandmother's inspiration – Nutripoints – and that by following its principles you may enjoy as full and as long a life as she did.

CONTENTS

FOREWORD

Nutrition for the 1990s will be more sophisticated, more scientific. No longer will we guess as to whether we are getting optimal nutrition; instead, we will measure it accurately.

In 1968 I developed a simple and easy-to-follow point system for exercise called 'aerobic' points. It revolutionized our concept of exercise. Now, at last, the same thing has been done for nutrition. A simple and easy-to-follow point system has been developed that, I predict, will permanently change the way we look at foods and nutrition.

After painstaking research and development using the Cooper Clinic Nutrition Database at the Aerobics Center, among others, Dr Roy Vartabedian has formulated the Nutripoint rating system. Nutripoints, based on nutrient density, quantifies precisely the quality of thousands of common foods by carefully comparing each food, nutrient by nutrient, to the American RDA (Recommended Daily Allowance) standards. In addition, the system adjusts for cholesterol, sodium, total and saturated fat, sugar, caffeine, and alcohol in each food. The result is one number that, taking into account all these factors, tells you the bottom line nutritional value of the food. I believe that Nutripoints will promote a major change in our Western diet, and will be an enormous help to everyone interested in avoiding the 'lifestyle' diseases – particularly heart disease and cancer.

A balanced programme for 'Total Well-Being' must include nutrition as its cornerstone. Nutripoints simplifies the complexities of nutrition with points to help you compare foods and track your progress. It's been used with tremendous success at the In-Residence Programs at the Aerobics Center and, I'm convinced that, coupled with an effective exercise programme, it can help you achieve a healthier, happier life!

Kenneth H. Cooper, M.D.

PART 1

Introduction

A word from Kathy Matthews:

The words 'revolutionary' and 'breakthrough' have become so commonplace these days that, when something that truly earns those descriptions comes along, we're left tongue tied. How *do* you describe a nutritional system that replaces counting calories*, worrying about fats, sugar and sodium, calculating cholesterol and working out RDAs (Recommended Daily Allowances) – a system that does all this and more with a simple number that tells you all you need to know to maintain a healthy diet?

Revolutionary, it certainly is.

A breakthrough, unquestionably.

In the same week that I met Dr Vartabedian, creator of Nutripoints, I received a frantic phone call from a friend. I've known Carol since college, and we've been through the diet wars together. About twenty pounds overweight, she had just decided to go on a simple, safe, low-calorie diet – one that I'm sure you've heard of. But she had also just visited her doctor who, because of her family medical history, had warned her that she must make a serious effort to get plenty of calcium in her diet. But he also warned her to avoid cholesterol-rich foods such as whole milk and dairy products. He said that the diet she planned was a good one, but she should be careful not to skimp on the recommended protein: adequate protein was essential if she wanted to lose weight safely and permanently.

Carol is vice president of a bank. She's motivated and intelligent and quite sophisticated about nutrition, but her head was spinning with her doctor's advice. 'Kathy,' she said on the phone, 'this isn't getting easier; it's getting harder. I want to lose weight but I don't want to have to become a professional dietitian. You've written two books on nutrition that were best-sellers. What can I eat?'

I promised to help Carol, but I knew that it would be a complicated and relatively tedious task. She needed high-quality protein that was

* **NB** strictly, *kilocalories*. However, *calorie* is used throughout the text as a shortened form for kilocalorie.

low in fat and cholesterol, and probably lots of green vegetables, some of which would help her get her calcium requirement. Would a grilled, skinless breast of chicken be a better choice than a grilled veal chop? And what about the days when I knew Carol had no time to cook . . . were there any frozen, prepared meals that were really good, nutritionally speaking? Was it really possible to get in a full day's nutrition – all the vitamins and minerals as well as adequate protein and carbohydrates – on a low-fat, low-calorie diet? When you came right down to it, what *were* the best foods to eat?

Carol's words rang in my ears and I realized that despite, or perhaps because of, the constant flood of nutritional information, finding your way through the food maze just wasn't becoming any easier.

And then I met Dr Vartabedian, a nutritional pioneer – really a visionary – who has assimilated all this contradictory data and gone one step beyond anyone in his field. Dr Vartabedian had already helped nearly 1,000 patients grappling with the same problems faced by my friend Carol. And like Carol, Dr Vartabedian's patients are intelligent, self-motivated readers of dozens of books and articles that have put them on a nutrition seesaw:

- this food is high in calcium, but also high in fat
- this food is low in fat, but high in sodium
- this food is high in protein, but also high in cholesterol
- this food is low in cholesterol, but high in saturated or 'bad' fat
- this food is low in calories but not very nutritious

When I recited the litany of seemingly contradictory nutritional recommendations that confuse us all, Dr Vartabedian acknowledged the confusion as the inspiration for Nutripoints. The following pages contain Dr Vartabedian's explanation of the Nutripoint concept and how it works.

'Update Overload' and the Confused Consumer

I think it is wonderful that updates of nutritional information have become fixtures in the news but, unfortunately, in my experience as a nutritionist who has seen thousands of patients over the course of my career, the real result of all this information is confusion. If a research finding doesn't help you in the kitchen or at the dining table, where it really counts, it can't do you any good.

When I was a student of nutrition, all of my questions about the body and the foods that fuel it were readily answered by my distinguished professors. Nutrition on the molecular level, while complicated, is relatively straightforward. It was only when I began to practise with actual patients that things became almost intolerably confusing, a confusion reflected in the case histories that follow:

- Mary had read in a women's magazine that if she didn't eat enough protein while trying to diet, she would lose muscle rather than fat and therefore regain any lost weight very quickly. But how much was enough protein? And didn't protein come mainly from meat and have a lot of fat? How could she find protein that didn't have a lot of calories?

- Roberta ate out in restaurants all the time. She knew the principles of good nutrition – avoid fried foods and creamy sauces, etc. – but what were the best and most healthy foods on a typical restaurant menu? Was tuna better or worse than baked plaice? What about a small, very lean roast pork chop compared to a few slices of lean boiled ham?

- James had suffered two heart attacks and was on a cholesterol lowering diet. However, he had to eat frequently at restaurants and just didn't know which foods – particularly meats – were the right ones to choose. He used to think that prawns were OK, but now he wasn't sure. Everything he read about cholesterol confused him even more.

- Ted called himself a 'businessman/athlete'. He jogged every morning and was in training for a local triathlon competition. He knew he needed to eat well, but he resorted to fast food all the time because he didn't enjoy cooking. Was he getting enough of the right kinds of foods? Was a Chicken à la King dinner that he could cook quickly in the microwave a good nutritional choice? How would it compare with, say, Gateway plaice fillets baked in crispy natural crumbs?

- Barbara had three children who were very fussy eaters. She knew that it was important for them to have proper nutrition in their growing years, but their eating habits were so erratic that she had no confidence that she was having any success. If they loved peanut butter and jam sandwiches, was that better or worse than a tuna sandwich? She avoided sugar in breakfast cereal but, aside from that, was one brand really better than another in terms of nutrition?

- Helen and her husband had retired, and faced many of the nutrition problems of the elderly: they had diminished appetites, and had to watch cholesterol carefully as well as fat intake. Because they were eating less, they had to be particularly careful to ensure adequate nutrition. Helen wanted to know if substitute foods were really OK to use. And would a vitamin pill take care of them on those days when they skipped a meal?

- Brian found himself eating at fast-food restaurants at least five times a week because they were quick and convenient. But what kind of nutrition was he getting from this sort of food? Was Kentucky fried chicken and chips better or worse than a Pizza Hut Pepperoni pan pizza? What were the *best* fast foods in terms of nutritional value?

These people came to me with their very real and pressing questions and I, as an expert, found it difficult to answer them. Most of us know what foods are 'good' for us; no one would argue that a carrot is 'good', as is an orange. And we also feel fairly comfortable pinpointing the 'bad' foods: fried bacon rind and fudge sauce would be picked out of any list of suspects by most people. But what about all those foods in between 'good' and 'bad'? How do you judge them? There was no gradient scale that could tell whether an apple was better than an orange or a fried bacon rind worse than a strip of fried bacon. Were there any dairy foods that were low in fat and at the same time high in calcium? Were high-fibre breakfast cereals or oat-bran breakfast cereals really good nutritional choices? Were some 'good' vegetables better than other 'good' vegetables?

These questions frustrated me as well as my patients. I realized that it was very easy to tell people what not to eat, but much harder to tell them what they should eat. The fact is that there's a whole spectrum of food values from very good to very bad, but there was no way to measure anything between those extremes. No one believed you could compare apples and oranges and no one had tried.

There was another factor involved as well. Suzanne put her finger on it for me when she came to see me about getting sufficient calcium in her pregnancy diet, while avoiding too many unnecessary calories (a very common question).

'Dr Vartabedian,' she complained, 'I'm really interested in nutrition and good food. And of course,' she gestured towards her growing waistline, 'never more so than now. But lately I've noticed that every time I think about food I feel anxious. Is it good for me? Good for the baby? Is it really nutritious? Does it have too much fat? Do embryos need to restrict their cholesterol intake?

'Sometimes I'm jealous of my mother who never worried about saturated fat in biscuits, and just ate what she wanted and tried not to eat too much. I read recently that stress increases your cholesterol levels. If that's true, it made me wonder if we aren't all taking one step forward and two steps back: we are so worried about how to eat healthily that even when we do eat the right things, our cholesterol levels are going up anyway from anxiety.'

Suzanne's feelings about food and eating had, over a period of years, gone from blithe unconcern – except for calories – to general anxiety: diet anxiety. She knew a lot about food, but she didn't know enough to put it all together.

Suzanne was an inspiration to me. Her words rang in my ears long after her healthy baby was born and I'd moved to a fascinating job at Dr Kenneth Cooper's Aerobics Center in Dallas. The Center offers the most comprehensive, state-of-the-art wellness programmes available in the world, and it gave me the opportunity to work with one of the most advanced nutritional data bases available. I knew that there must be a solution to Suzanne's dilemma – diet anxiety – and I set out to find it.

Over the course of years, working with hundreds of patients, I finally refined a system that I believe answers all of today's perplexing nutritional questions. It's a system that not only tells you which foods are good and which are bad, it also establishes a gradient scale that measures all foods. And not only does it rate all foods, it provides a simple system that gives you an optimally balanced diet, one that allows you the luxury of choice.

Nutripoints is my answer for all the patients whose questions I have so painstakingly answered after much labour. Nutripoints is the tool that will allow them, and anyone else interested in good nutrition, to find an optimum diet.

We should not be confused about food. Above all, we should not be anxious about what we eat. My hope is that Nutripoints will be a giant step towards returning us to safe, pleasurable, healthy eating.

The Nutripoints Revolution

The Nutripoints Programme is something very different from anything you've come across. It is an actual nutritional advance and a quantum leap in our ability to eat a healthy diet. It will provide you with a completely new approach to eating. Here are the four revolutionary features of the Nutripoints Programme that make it so effective and appealing:

● *Nutripoints is the only nutritional information you'll ever need.*

Nutripoints guarantees that you meet and exceed all the major international nutritional guidelines regarding daily intakes of every major nutrient including protein, carbohydrates, fibre, vitamins and minerals, while at the same time staying well below the allowable levels of fat, cholesterol, sugar and sodium.

Have you ever stood in the supermarket trying to work out what grams of fat mean in terms of calories? Have you ever wondered what it means when a packaged food provides 100 per cent of your daily requirements of one vitamin and 0 per cent of everything else? Have you been on diets that you later learned were damaging to your health, even though they might be effective? Do you get confused about whether skimmed or semi-skimmed milk is better for you in terms of fat content? And do you know which cheeses are lowest in cholesterol?

Before Nutripoints, you would have had to do twenty-six different mathematical calculations on each food you eat to have only the *basis* for the information Nutripoints gives in one number.

Now you can forget about calories and grams of fat and milligrams of sodium – and even forget about reading nutritional labels. And you don't have to abandon hope totally when you eat in a fast-food restaurant. Nutripoints weighs *all* the bad factors in a food against *all* the good factors, and comes up with a simple number that tells you all you need to know to provide the human machine with the best possible fuel.

For example, imagine you're choosing fruit juices. Here is a small sample of the Nutripoint ratings for juices:

Juice	Nutripoints
Fresh squeezed orange juice	11.5
Reconstituted frozen orange juice	11.0
Unsweetened grapefruit juice	11.0
Sweetened grapefruit juice	7.0
Unsweetened grape juice	5.5
Apple juice	2.5

A quick glance at this chart tells you that sweetened grapefruit juice is not nearly as good as orange juice. And apple juice is only fractionally as good as fresh or frozen orange juice. The Nutripoint charts make it easy to choose a juice that you and your family like, as well as a juice that provides good nutrition.

Now let's say that you're choosing a cereal. Here are the numbers for just a few:

Cereal	Nutripoints
Kellogg's All Bran	27.0
Nabisco 100% Bran Cereal	23.5
Kellogg's Corn Flakes	18.0
Kellogg's Special K	14.0
Weetabix	6.5
Lyons' Ready Brek	6.0
RHM Shredded Wheat	5.0

The general trend with cereals is that as more sugar and processing come into play and the original whole food, if any, is adulterated, the lower the level of nutrition. Consequently, cereals scoring high on the scale contain more bran or whole grain as well as less sugar (and possibly more added vitamins) than the others. Once again, if you're concerned with good nutrition, you need only look for the high numbers to find the best choices.

Whether you're choosing between broccoli or Brussels sprouts; plaice or salmon; cheddar or goat's cheese; or even between chocolate bars, Nutripoints is your good-food bible.

- *Nutripoints is the first positive approach to nutrition that eliminates rigid adhesion to menus and meal plans, because the balance is 'built in'.*

Any diet in the past has had to rely on various meal plans that sometimes became very complicated. That's because there was no other way to ensure that people would get the correct balance of foods. You can't just eat low-calorie foods and be well nourished: you need to eat from a broad spectrum of foods. The best diets were well constructed: someone worked out how much fat, protein, complex carbohydrates, etc. was in each food and each meal, and then made sure that these amounts were adequate. But you had to follow a very specific daily menu plan or a complicated system of 'substitutions' in order to maintain the nutritional balance. Nutripoints makes that rigid approach redundant, because it provides a *comprehensive system* that allows you to create your own meal plans. By following the recommendations concerning numbers of servings from the six Nutrigroups, you'll be guaranteed an optimum diet – one of your own choosing.

The Nutripoints Programme is totally flexible. Once you're familiar with Nutripoints, you need only focus on the foods you like and the foods that are readily available to you to create meals that give you the best possible nutritional value. You won't be shopping for fish to grill on a day that you're really in the mood for some kind of pasta or rice dish.

Once you're familiar with Nutripoints, you'll find it will become an instinctive way of eating. Best of all, you'll find that simply by choosing your foods from the top of the Nutripoint charts, and getting the recommended servings from every Nutrigroup, you'll be getting a higher daily intake of every single vitamin and mineral, as well as the optimum amount of fibre, protein, carbohydrates and fat. You'll also be limiting your total fat, saturated fat, cholesterol, sugar, sodium, caffeine and alcohol.

Hundreds of Nutripoint converts agree that it's the best remedy for diet anxiety.

● *Nutripoints not only lets you know what's bad; it separates the very best from the good.*

Most foods have some bad things in them as well as some good. But how much bad and how much good? How do you evaluate this difference? Dairy foods seem to be particularly confusing today, because of the very real concern about calcium. Everyone knows they need to get adequate calcium, but the foods that are very high in calcium – like milk and cheese – are also very high in fat. Nutripoints eliminates the confusion. The higher the Nutripoint score, the lower in fat *and* the higher in calcium of the rated food. Evaluating the crucial differences in foods is what Nutripoints is all about.

Here's an illustration of how Nutripoints shows how processing lowers the score on a particular food.

Food	Nutripoints
potato, baked	8.5
potatoes au gratin	2.5
scalloped potatoes	2.0
mashed potatoes, home recipe	1.0
French fries	1.0
potato crisps	0.0
potato salad, home recipe	– 1.0

You can readily see that the more a food is processed, the more salt and fatty substances are added, the more the original vitamin and mineral content is tampered with, the lower its Nutripoints.

Do you like yogurt? Do you think it's good for you? Here are the facts:

Yogurt	Nutripoints
Very low fat Shape strawberry yogurt	10.5
St Ivel low fat natural yogurt	8.0
Chambourcy B'Active set yogurt	4.5

Sainsbury's natural set yogurt	3.0
Ski low fat raspberry yogurt	2.5
Greek cow's yogurt	0.0

As the fat and the sugar go up, the Nutripoints go down. Your yogurt choice is between an excellent serving of very low fat yogurt (with fresh fruit added to boost your Nutripoints score) or, say, Greek yogurt, which you may think is good for you but which actually does you little nutritional good.

But there are factors other than processing – factors in the food itself that affect its Nutripoint score. Indeed, if you're someone who pays attention to good nutrition and tries to eat well, you will no doubt find that Nutripoints is the first system that tells you something that you don't already know. Here's an example. If you thought that simple steamed prawns was a good diet food – low in calories but high in protein – you'll be interested to learn that 15 medium prawns earn only 0.5 Nutripoints while 3 oz (75 g) baked or grilled salmon is worth 5.5 Nutripoints, eleven times the nutritional value. If you've been starving yourself on occasions, thinking that a lunch of a few prawns and some lettuce is a virtuous choice, you will be delighted to learn that you're really better off with a salmon (mixed with yogurt and vegetables) sandwich made with wholemeal bread. You'll be more full, you'll be better nourished and, if losing weight is your goal, you'll be better served.

Most of us know we should cut down on fat. But knowing these things isn't much help when it comes down to shopping and eating. Nutripoints to the rescue: For example, did you know that Quark soft skimmed milk cheese (at 9.5 Nutripoints) is a great substitute for Philadelphia full fat soft cheese (at – 5.5 Nutripoints) when you want something to spread on a roll?

Many people have abandoned tinned fruit, thinking that only fresh was of any merit, but in fact 4 oz (100 g) of tinned mandarin orange slices without sugar has a Nutripoint value of 15.5 while a *fresh* pear earns only 4.5 Nutripoints. Mandarin oranges simply have more nutrition – more Vitamin C and more fibre than a fresh pear.

What about a soup for a quick lunch? Heinz Chicken and Mushroom at – 4.0 Nutripoints isn't the great nutritional bargain we might have expected, but Lentil with Ham at 4.5 Nutripoints is a good alternative. And what about those evenings when you don't have a minute to spare – chicken breast baked without skin at 4.0 Nutripoints or baked haddock fillet at 5.0 Nutripoints are both quick, nutritious meals. But the Tesco's frozen Shepherd's pie at 0.0 Nutripoints or fish fingers at 0.5 Nutripoints are not nutritional bargains.

If you're like most of my patients, just a glance at the Nutripoints food lists will be both a revelation for you and a revolution for your future diet.

- *Nutripoints is the only nutritional system that allows for recovery from 'being bad'.*

We've become so chained to the 'calories per day' or 'fat per day' notion of nutrition that it's a relief to substitute the Nutripoints concept which deals with *real* nutrition in the real world. The fact is that, in terms of nutrition, a day is a very short time-frame. For example, your body stores Vitamin A for weeks. With the Nutripoints Programme you no longer have to think about a twenty-four-hour make-it-or-break-it eating pattern: you can spread things out over the course of a few days. Though, for the sake of convenience, you'll still be aiming for a daily total of 100 points, you can be flexible enough to go over or under on any given day and make up for the lack within another day or two.

Because Nutripoints gives you a way of measuring the values of the foods you eat, it gives you an opportunity to get back on track if you fall behind.

Nutripoints is such a simple 'numbers game' with negative and positive numbers that, if you have a really bad day in which you eat the wrong foods (a day with a negative total of Nutripoints), you can still end up with an excellent nutritional week.

This expansion of the basic diet time-frame removes one of the most persistent and discouraging psychological barriers to effective dieting – the old 'I've blown it today so I might as well forget it' rationale.

Future Foods

You're probably aware that the foods you eat are very different from those eaten by your grandparents. What determines how 'food styles' change? Agricultural trends, food storage and distribution methods all have some effect, but a big determinant is simple fashion. It's no longer fashionable, for example, for a woman or man to display their wealth with their girth. It made cultural sense, once upon a time, to achieve status with the evidence of rich and lavish meals. The lean and hungry peasant would look with longing at the tubby Lord. Today that trend is fully reversed: for years now people have believed that you can never be too thin or too rich.

In addition to fashion, there are practical reasons for a changing diet. A farmer, faced with a day of hard physical labour from sunrise to sunset, is going to have nutritional needs that differ substantially from those of a stockbroker or a bank clerk. The latter simply don't need the greater amounts of fuel required by a body that's doing hard labour.

The great nutritional challenge we face today can be stated simply: our optimum diet has two principles that seem diametrically opposed – we need to get high levels of nutrients (to keep our bodies functioning well while helping them to fight the effects of disease, ageing and pollution), and we need to achieve this in fewer and fewer calories (to avoid excess weight that affects our appearance and our health).

These needs force us to scrutinize our foods in a new way. If we want to achieve optimum health and longevity we have to think about *nutrients per calorie*.

Nutrients per calorie is the basic cost/benefit analysis we have to keep in mind when we choose foods. It's analogous to our efforts to get the best value for money when buying a product. Because we are usually limiting our calorie intake, every single calorie has to count in terms of overall nutritional value. Here's an example: there is ample Vitamin C in half an avocado, but it will 'cost' 160 calories, while a glass of grapefruit juice has nine times the Vitamin C of the avocado at a 'cost' of only 95 calories.

The concept of nutrients per calorie explains why junk foods are junk: they provide virtually no nutrition and a lot of calories. Take, for example, a typical fast-food lunch: a Big Mac with a large order of fries and a Coke. This meal gives you only 30–50 per cent of your major nutrients at a cost of 1,064 calories. For many people that's the *total* number of calories they should have in a day – and they haven't even consumed *half* their necessary nutrients. With Nutripoints, you can get more than your daily allowance of minerals and vitamins along with the optimum amounts of fibre, protein, and complex carbohydrates, with the *same* number of calories.

You must remember, also, that it costs vitamins and minerals to burn up calories. If you're not getting adequate nutrients along with the calories you're burning up, the body's stores of vitamins and minerals must be called upon to make up for the lack in the food itself. This is the damaging but very common predicament that can lead to clinical or sub-clinical deficiencies and less-than-optimal functioning of various body processes.

A high nutrient-per-calorie ratio is the basic principle of every healthy diet. Nutripoints rates every food on the basis of this crucial nutrient-per-calorie ratio. Moreover, because Nutripoints lists all kinds of food, it allows you to create your own diet – one that suits *your* tastes and *your* lifestyle.

The Nutripoint Numbers

Nutripoints is a very simple way of dealing with something very complex. It is a number system for rating foods.

The Nutripoints programme has four important principles:

1 *Nutripoint values*

Each food has a given Nutripoint value. It is amazingly simple: the higher the Nutripoint score of a given food, the higher in the 'good' components of foods (including all the important vitamins and minerals and fibre and protein), and the lower in the 'bad' components (including calories, cholesterol, total fat, saturated fat, sodium, sugar, caffeine and alcohol). A large variety of foods, including basic foods, processed foods, fast foods, and even 'health' foods, has been evaluated and assigned a number.

Some foods fall below a 'not recommended' level and some foods are so low in Nutripoints that they have negative Nutripoint values. However, Nutripoint values are provided for many foods, even poor nutritional choices. This is the way in which Nutripoints differs from typical diets. *Foods are evaluated in terms of Nutripoints.* This allows you to compare the bad with the good, as well as the good with the best.

A glance at the Nutripoints for various foods is an eye-opener. For instance, we all know the old adage about 'an apple a day . . .', but did you know that melon is a far better choice? In the fruit Nutrigroup, although both are 'good' for you, a quarter of a cantaloupe melon has 29 Nutripoints whereas an apple has only 4.5. The melon has fewer calories (40 versus 50 for the apple) and more iron, fifty times the Vitamin A, ten times the Vitamin C, more folic acid, thiamin, more riboflavin and more of virtually every other nutrient. Raw spinach at 75 Nutripoints is a much better vegetable than plain iceberg lettuce at 18.0 Nutripoints, even though both are low in calories!

Many people are surprised to learn that some cuts of lean beef are better choices than some types of fish. For example, lean round steak at 4.0 Nutripoints is a better choice than baked plaice at 3.5 Nutripoints. And broccoli, at 38.5 Nutripoints, is terrific nutritional value compared with a baked potato at 8.5 Nutripoints.

As I mentioned, there are negative Nutripoints and there's also a cut-off point below which foods are not recommended. The numbers are interesting just as a basis of comparison between foods, but you also need them to work out your daily Nutripoint scores.

2 Nutripoint quotas

Of course the numbers assigned to foods have to be put into a workable context: what do they really add up to? You can't just eat a few servings of spinach a day and get a lot of Nutripoints and consider yourself well nourished. There has to be a balance of different kinds of foods over a period of time.

The Nutripoints Programme recommends that you get 100 Nutripoints per day. Not only will you get the necessary amounts of eighteen important nutrients, you will at the same time limit the calories, sugar, cholesterol, total fat, saturated fat, sodium, caffeine and alcohol in your diet, and in one easy step help prevent and control heart disease, hypertension, diabetes, obesity, osteoporosis, cancer and other lifestyle diseases.

Of course, 100 Nutripoints is just a basic goal: you may fall below it on some days and exceed it by a wide margin on others. Here's a chart that will show you how you can assess a daily Nutripoints score:

Daily Nutripoint scores

25   – very poor
50   – poor
75   – fair
100   – good
150   – excellent
200 + – superior

3 *Nutripoint balance*

In order for the Nutripoints Programme to work, your diet must be balanced. You can't eat 3 oz (75 g) turnip tops (39.5 Nutripoints), some asparagus (44 Nutripoints), some raw radishes (29 Nutripoints), and some cucumber (20 Nutripoints) for a total of 103.5 Nutripoints, and then call it a day. You have to choose from different food groups to be sure that you cover all your nutritional bases.

There are six basic Nutrigroups. To achieve the Nutripoint balance, you must achieve a Nutripoint goal for each group and *you must do it within the recommended number of servings*. The serving quota is a limiting device: you want to score the highest possible number of Nutripoints, but you can't do it by simply eating enormous quantities of one food!

Here's a simple breakdown of the food-group system:

The daily Nutripoint recommendations

Servings	Nutrigroup	Nutripoints
4	vegetables	55
3	fruits	15
2	grains	10
1	pulses/nuts/seeds	5
2	milk/dairy	10
1	meat/poultry/fish	5
	Total	100

Here's what the chart means to you on a daily basis. You need to ensure that you get 4 vegetable servings daily. Many vegetables are very high in Nutripoints, and I think you'll find it quite easy to get 55 points per day. For example, you might have a tossed salad (33 Nutripoints) at lunch, broccoli (38.5 Nutripoints) and a baked potato (8.5) at dinner, and a glass of carrot juice (15.0 Nutripoints) as a snack. This would give you your 4 vegetable servings for a total of 95.0 Nutripoints – well above the 55 Nutripoints you're supposed to get from the vegetable group.

Of course, now and again you may have a day where you don't do very well at all. Perhaps you'll have a three bean salad (1.5), some French fries (1.0 Nutripoints), some cooked courgettes (15 Nutripoints) and some sweet pickle (0.5 Nutripoints). Your total vegetable score on that day is 18 Nutripoints from your 4 servings from the vegetable Nutrigroup. You can boost your score with good choices from the other groups. And you can boost your long-term score with the Nutripoint Recovery . . .

4 Nutripoint Recovery

What does it really mean if you get more or fewer than 100 Nutripoints daily? It's an opportunity to see your nutritional status in terms of more than just one day.

Most diets are limited to a one-day pattern which, for many dieters, means a nutritional tightrope – if you weaken and have some barbecued chicken at a party, the day is lost. This is enormously discouraging. Even if the diet tells you to view the lapse as a mistake and to move on from there, you're never given a method that allows you to incorporate the mistake into the diet plan.

Nutripoints is the first and only nutritional system that gives you an opportunity for recovery! Nutripoints, which is really a leap beyond 'dieting', gives you the flexibility to 'recover' from a lapse. You no longer have to despair about a bad day.

While you're aiming for 100 Nutripoints per day, the Nutripoints Programme allows you to quantify the values of the foods you're eating and thereby 'make up' for a bad day within the next day or two. If you have a business dinner that includes a high-fat French meal that plunges your Nutripoints to a negative number, you can boost your scores back up to optimal levels with some high Nutripoint scores during the next few days. So if your French débâcle day totals 32 Nutripoints, you can go for the gold for the next two days, trying to get well in excess of your recommended daily 100 points.

The important point is that because Nutripoints gives you a way of *measuring* the value of your nutritional intake, it also gives you a method of recovering from losses. You cannot 'bank' Nutripoints: you can't prepare for a binge on Wednesday by getting high scores on Monday and Tuesday. After all, you're fooling no one but yourself if you try to use Nutripoints in that way. But you don't have to feel defeated by a day's low score.

And, let's face it, not all our lapses are forced. What about when you're just dying for an ice-cream cone? Or what if you eat chocolate gateaux? With the Nutripoint System you have a method of atonement. You only need to ensure that you make up for those negative points within a couple of days.

I want to emphasize that Nutripoints does not 'encourage' or even 'allow for' regular diet lapses. It just doesn't make nutritional sense to try to eat well most of the time but, say, twice a week, have a small binge. The Nutripoints Programme assumes that you're serious about good nutrition. It simply recognizes that there will be occasions when you'll eat something that isn't of good nutritional value. There's no sense in pretending this doesn't happen, so Nutripoints takes it into consideration and incorporates it into the system.

This recovery feature of Nutripoints has been one that patients have found very reassuring. Many studies have shown that 'restrained eaters' who are severely limited in the type or amount of food they can eat will eventually binge or relapse. Nutripoints provides powerful psychological motivation because it allows you to 'make up' for lapses. It's also far more realistic to assume that people will have good and bad days: Nutripoints gives you a framework that takes real life into consideration.

The extraordinary benefit of Nutripoints is that, if you've adopted the nutritional goals of the Nutripoints Programme, you will probably be better nourished than you've ever been in your life, even if you have a bad day!

Nutripoints in the Real World

It's one thing to come up with the best all-round system for evaluating foods. But the best and most sophisticated charts in the world won't help people if they don't or can't use them. Nutripoints' track record for changing people's lives is convincing evidence that it's a system that's easy to live with, no matter what your lifestyle.

Here's the story of Jane, a Nutripoint convert who came to the system reluctantly. I want to tell you about Jane because, while some patients have experienced more dramatic changes in their overall health profile, Jane illustrates two elements of Nutripoints:

1 It's incredibly easy to live with.
2 It's valuable even for people who think that their diet is already nutritionally sound.

Jane is the 42-year-old manager of a corporate health programme for a large national company. Her job gives her reason and opportunity to keep up with the latest medical advances and theories, but she's also personally interested. When the time came for her company to make an arrangement with a 'corporate health centre' to do complete check-ups on their employees, Jane became a 'guinea pig' so that she could acquire a good understanding of the services offered by the centre.

Though Jane hadn't had a complete physical examination for some years, she had no complaints that she considered serious, or even worthy of mention. She often had a headache in the afternoon, and she was usually exhausted after work, but she thought that these symptoms had more to do with her demanding schedule than anything else. Though she counselled employees to take regular exercise, Jane herself was sedentary except for an occasional game of tennis in the summer. She knew that she should lose about 10 or perhaps 15 pounds in weight, but she thought that her diet was pretty good except for the regular business lunches when she found it impossible to eat lightly. All in all, Jane thought she was healthy and didn't expect any surprises from her check-up.

But when the print-out from the health centre arrived, Jane was shocked. Her cholesterol was 228 (5.5 mmol/l), her blood pressure was slightly elevated, her 15 pounds of excess weight was confirmed, and her treadmill time which measured her aerobic endurance level was terrible. Still worse, her family history of osteoporosis indicated that she'd have to increase her calcium intake dramatically but, because of her cholesterol and her excess weight, she'd have to be especially careful to avoid fat. She also had a family history of breast cancer, and the latest evidence showed that a reduction in her fat intake would be imperative if she wanted to improve her chances of avoiding this disease.

Because of her work in the health field, Jane had heard about the Cooper Aerobics Center and she enrolled in our four-day Aerobics Wellness Weekend. When she arrived, she told me that the results of her physical examination had really overwhelmed her; it was the first time she'd felt really 'mortal', as she put it. And she was also confused. Though she knew what her dietary goals should be, she didn't know how to achieve them. She hated the idea of a typical diet, because she really didn't believe that she'd be able to keep to one. But she felt she needed a 'crash course' on nutrition to get her on track. She was very frank when she told me that she didn't expect to change her life; she just wanted to 'pick my brains' to learn what she should be eating and then she'd go about things her own way. But she warned me not to expect her to stick with an eating programme once she was back on her home territory.

I began by giving Jane a brief explanation of the Nutripoints Programme. She was fascinated by the numbers, and eager to see how they'd apply to her own life. I asked Jane to chart a typical day's eating. She felt she was on solid ground here. She was convinced that her diet was excellent. Here is what she came up with:

Breakfast	Nutripoints
English whole wheat muffin (no butter)	6.0
coffee	− 3.5
cream (non-dairy)	− 3.5
Snack	
1 container fruits of the forest yogurt	1.5
Lunch	
tuna noodle casserole	3.5
bread	2.5

butter	− 6.5
1 glass wine	− 13.0
salad	33.0
Italian dressing	− 2.5

Dinner

chicken pot pie	0.5
frozen yogurt	1.5
2 glasses wine	− 26.0
Total	− 6.5

Jane said that on some days she ate much more and on others less, but this was a fairly typical meal pattern. She thought it was pretty good – after all, she didn't eat much meat or any eggs and she tried to avoid sweets. The fact is that Jane's total daily Nutripoint score was − 6.5! Even if you forget about the wine she drank, which dramatically lowered her score, you're left with a score of 32.5. This is a dismal score – particularly when you bear in mind that Jane thought of herself as someone who was well versed in nutrition!

It's shocking when you become familiar with Nutripoints and when your sense of what constitutes good nutrition changes, but Jane's diet was typical of someone who knew a fair amount about nutrition in the 1980s. She knew to avoid certain fats and sweets and, of course, that's good. But she had no notion about the *positive* elements that she was missing in her diet. And she was also eating lots of *hidden* fats and sweets. Jane was really short-changing herself and her body was beginning to show the symptoms.

Because Jane was so resistant to a 'diet', I decided to ease her into the Nutripoints Programme. I told her we'd stick with her typical eating pattern, but we'd *upgrade* it with Nutripoints. Here's Jane's typical day on Nutripoints:

Breakfast

Kellogg's corn flakes	18.0
skimmed milk	5.0
¼ cantaloupe melon	29.0
coffee	− 3.5
skimmed milk	0.5

Snack

plain very low fat yogurt	8.5
frozen strawberries	17.0

Lunch

lentil soup	5.5
macaroni with beef and tomato sauce	3.0
bread (no butter)	2.5
tossed salad	33.0
yogurt dressing	0.5
fresh fruit salad	13.0

Dinner

Tesco's sliced turkey breast	6.5
Bird's Eye frozen broccoli, cauliflower, red peppers	41.5
Sainsbury's strawberry very low fat yogurt	10.0
Total	180.0

Jane couldn't believe that she was eating almost exactly the same things she'd been eating before and yet improving her diet by about 150 per cent! A few simple tricks improved her Nutripoint score dramatically. For example, she found that it was no trouble to put some frozen berries in a cup of very low fat yogurt in the morning before she left for work. The berries helped keep the yogurt cold and by the time she was ready for her snack, they were defrosted. She says the 'fruit added' yogurt now tastes sickeningly sweet to her. After three days at the Center eating similar meals that I had devised for her based on her own preferences, Jane was a convert.

After two months on Nutripoints, Jane phoned me to tell me the results of her latest physical examination. She'd returned to the corporate health centre to get an update and she was delighted with the news: her cholesterol was 186 (4.9 mmol/l), down 18 per cent; her weight was down 12 pounds; and her blood pressure was completely normal.

Jane was quick to tell me that she didn't stick religiously to the Programme. Every now and again she slipped, but not because she wanted to. It was always because she found herself in a situation –

usually a social one like a dinner party – where it was almost impossible to stick with her new patterns. For example, her worst day included a dinner party at the home of a business colleague. She had two glasses of dry white wine (at – 14 Nutripoints each), a crabmeat salad with hollandaise sauce (at – 6.0 Nutripoints), chicken Kiev (at 0.0 Nutripoints), a salad with blue cheese dressing (at 30 Nutripoints) and German chocolate cake (at – 3.5 Nutripoints). Even though Jane tried to sample only some of the dishes she thought were the worst Nutripoint values, she still found herself with a score of – 7.5 Nutripoints for that meal. As she said, 'The cook has spent an enormous amount of time and trouble to plunge me into negative Nutripoints!' On the day of that dinner, Jane's Nutripoints came to 53. But she was only more resolved to make up for the loss and go for the top of the list for the rest of the week. And she did it!

Why Nutripoints Could Be *Your* Nutritional Breakthrough

One morning, not too long ago, the phone rang in my office. It was Richard, a computer artist who had visited the Aerobics Center two months previously with his wife. Richard had made the visit for his wife's sake, but he had no real interest in participating. As Richard was extremely overweight and extremely reluctant to try any kind of diet, I was surprised to hear from him. By the time he left the Aerobics Center I believed that he had a psychological problem that was preventing him from making an effort; psychology is not my field, but when you work with people who are trying to change their lives, you learn something about what makes them tick.

'Dr Vartabedian,' Richard said, 'I have a confession to make. When I got home from the Aerobics Center I was angry. I suppose I really believed that if I paid the money to be there it would *have* to help me. Yes, I was there for my wife's sake, but I also wondered if the visit could really help me too. But I almost had a chip on my shoulder about it.

'I guess because I didn't have any success, I'm ashamed to say that I made fun of the food charts my wife was using. She was making real progress and I suppose I just couldn't take it. Well, a week after I got home I found myself standing at the refrigerator eating raw chocolate chip cookie dough right out of the roll by the spoonful. By the time I had finished half the roll, I felt awful – dizzy and light-headed. I went to lie down and, as I stretched out on the couch, I thought, really thought, about what I had done. I was so disgusted with myself that I wasn't sure which was making me sicker: the cookie dough or my own behaviour. I decided to give Nutripoints a try. I knew I couldn't change overnight, but I remembered enough about what you'd said about Nutripoints to know that I could do it at my own pace. And I wanted to thank you because, as of today, I've lost 21 pounds. I also wanted to tell you that it's the only thing that's ever worked for me. The only reason that it's worked is because it's really easy. I have a long way to go but for the first time in my life, I know I'm going to get there.'

I'm telling Richard's story because he illustrates what I think is the most important feature of Nutripoints: it's easy. Though many people want to improve their lives, they find it just too difficult without major motivation. I believe that's because diet and exercise pro- grammes are just too difficult. They're not fun: they're grim and they make you feel like a penitent. They demand major changes and they demand that you give up patterns and habits that may have taken a lifetime to acquire. So most people never experience the pleasure of a body enjoying optimum nutrition or anything near it.

If you want to improve your nutrition but are discouraged by difficult diets with complicated menus, the Nutripoints Programme will change your life. One of my goals in developing Nutripoints was to find something that *everyone* – even people who would never follow a typical diet – would find readily accessible.

Here are the features that I think will make the difference for you. First, you'll find that it's the simplest and most positive approach to nutrition you've ever encountered. If you like, you can ease into it: just use the charts to improve the quality of everything you eat. Focus on the positive and you'll soon find yourself avoiding the negative too. I've seen many people ease their way into the system with great success. Maria is an example. She came to our 13-Day Aerobics Program for Total Well-Being at the Aerobics Center with her husband, who was showing early signs of heart disease. She was there only to offer moral support; she exercised regularly and, though she would have liked to lose a few pounds, she didn't want to 'diet'. As she now says, 'Once I realized that I could lose a bit of weight and dramatically improve the quality of my diet simply by making some informed comparisons of foods and eliminating a few foods that tipped the balance the wrong way, I couldn't *help* but do it. My nutritional status was not great. I was eating bad stuff and I suppose, without realizing it, I was on a gradual decline. You just don't stop and see what you're doing to yourself day to day.

'I never would have thought about making a change without Nutripoints. It never occurred to me before Nutripoints just why typical reducing or health-oriented diets turned me off. They all seemed to be complicated or offer a gimmick that I couldn't really believe in. But Nutripoints is not really a diet; it's a *tool* based on real science that allows you to go as far as you want to improve your nutrition. My husband has certainly changed his life and dramatically improved his health – his cholesterol is already down 46 points (approx. 1 mmol/l) – but I always felt convinced that would happen if he made major changes in his diet. The real surprise is me. I never would have believed that I'd jump on the Nutripoint bandwagon and, given the fact that I didn't think I needed any improvement, I'm amazed at the changes I see in me and my husband. I've lost those few extra pounds and the general improvement in the way both my husband and I feel is really wonderful. We've got more energy, we're more calm. We feel just great.'

There's a second, bonus benefit to Nutripoints: you won't have to wait years to enjoy its effects. Here are the average changes experienced by patients at the 13-day Aerobics Program for Total Well-Being:

weight	8 lbs (3.2 kg) or 4% decrease
serum cholesterol	14% decrease
serum cholesterol-HDL ratio*	16% decrease
serum glucose	10% decrease
serum triglycerides	
(other blood fats)	40% decrease
treadmill time (fitness level)	19% increase
blood pressure	6% decrease

Now these patients are working on exercise and stress reduction in addition to nutrition. But if you undertake the Nutripoints Programme with any measure of seriousness, and you work on stress reduction and exercise too, there's no reason why you can't experience similar improvements. And, from a more short-term point of view, you'll probably experience freedom from digestive problems, sluggishness, inability to concentrate, frequent headaches and irritability. And in mid-afternoon, when many people start to fade, you'll find that you have the energy and stamina to keep going.

* Cholesterol levels can be measured in two ways: total cholesterol measures all types found in the blood whereas high-density cholesterol (HDL) refers to good, protective cholesterol only. The higher the HDL is in relation to total cholesterol, the better.

PART 2

The Science of
Optimal Nutrition

'Scared Smart'

For a moment, forget pills, forget exercise, forget relaxation techniques. The simple fact is that the single most important step you can take today to improve your overall sense of well-being and your long-term health is to improve your nutrition. Exercise works the body; food *makes* the body. There are many billions of cells in your body, and each one is made up of and nourished by the food you eat. You simply can't function at your best, as we'll see, if you don't eat the best foods. Of course, exercise, stress-reduction techniques and all sensible efforts at better health make sense. But if you don't improve your nutrition, your other efforts will be well-nigh pointless.

Does it really matter that you keep your fat, cholesterol and sodium levels down? That you make a point of getting all the vitamins and minerals your body needs? I'm so used to dealing with the educated demands of my patients at the Aerobics Center that I sometimes forget that anyone today needs convincing.

The people who come to me for help with their diets are highly motivated. In many cases, 'motivated' is a euphemism for 'terrified'. Some of my patients are actually staring death in the face. They've suffered a heart attack, maybe two. I think of these people as 'scared smart'. They have decided they want to live, and they're prepared to do anything it takes to make that happen. The Nutripoints Programme is an enormous relief to them; it's an eating programme that will help them literally to save their own lives. In addition, it is easy to incorporate into their lifestyles and it allows them to devise their own eating programmes: many of these people believed that they would have to live on a terribly restricted, boring diet for the rest of their lives.

I hope that the majority of the rest of us – the lucky ones who haven't been forced to change our diets because of illness – have moved out of the Dark Ages of Nutrition where we believed we could eat whatever we wanted, and trust to luck or good genes to get us through. It just doesn't work that way; it really is up to you.

Cholesterol was the red flag that alerted millions of people to the fact that diet really does matter – that what we're eating every day is going to make a difference to how we feel both today and tomorrow. But cholesterol is only part of the story. Today, largely because of diet, a very significant proportion of the population are at risk from heart disease, diabetes, hypertension and cancer. The American Cancer Society recently announced that they expected 1 million Americans to have a cancer diagnosis in 1989 – the first time the projection has reached that mark. In addition to the over 1 million new cancer cases, the Society projected over half a million cancer deaths for that year. A well-documented percentage of cancers – only one of the leading causes of death – are diet related.

It's no news that the Western diet can be dangerous to your health. In 1977 George McGovern headed a congressional committee that investigated the long-term effects of what Americans eat. The McGovern committee studied the relationship between this diet and the nation's major killers – heart disease, cancers of the colon and breast, stroke, high blood pressure, obesity, diabetes, arteriosclerosis, and cirrhosis of the liver. They estimated that if Americans modified their rich diets, there would be an 80 per cent drop in the number of obese people, a 25 per cent drop in deaths from heart disease, a 50 per cent drop in deaths from diabetes and a 1 per cent annual increase in longevity.

It seems that every day there's a new study that demonstrates the dangers of fats and cholesterol and the importance of fibre and various nutrients such as calcium in the diet. A recent study confirmed yet again the dangers for women of a high-calorie, high-fat diet. This study overwhelmingly demonstrated that women who ate the most fats, saturated fats and animal protein had a three times greater chance of getting breast cancer than those whose intake of these foods was lowest. Moreover, it showed that a high-calorie diet made women almost twice as likely to develop breast cancer.

The connections between a diet high in fat and cholesterol and calories have been definitively linked to the major lifestyle diseases. The answer couldn't be more obvious: if you want to avoid the major killing and debilitating diseases, improve your diet.

Beyond Calories

How *do* you improve your diet? Well, you try to cut down on fat and cholesterol and probably calories . . . But how do you actually go about doing this? The first thing you do is discard your old notions about how to judge foods. If you're like most people, the calorie is the only food measure that you're really familiar with. It's time to forget calories and move on to Nutripoints.

To understand just how revolutionary Nutripoints is, you need only take a look at what has existed in the past to help people choose among foods.

We are all calorie 'nuts'. We have some notion that we have to have variety – something about choosing from different food groups – but counting calories has been the most common system for comparing foods. Most people who pay attention to what they eat are trying to lose weight. They look for foods that are low in calories. But we now know that calories are just one measure of the value of various foods. A diet extremely low in calories can also be a diet that is nutritionally unsound – sometimes even dangerous, as we've seen from some fad diets. And a diet extremely low in calories is not necessarily a diet that will promote permanent weight loss.

The RDAs – the Recommended Daily Allowances – provide a standard by which food can be measured. The US figures were arrived at by the Food and Nutrition Board, a committee of the National Academy of Sciences-National Research Council. The RDAs used in the UK were determined by the Committee on Medical Aspects of Food Policy. As in the US the RDAs are supposed to be 'the levels of intake of essential nutrients considered to be adequate to meet the known nutritional needs of practically all healthy persons'.

Nutritional information is provided on many foods, though of course unprocessed foods don't provide the convenient labels that would help you determine whether a white or a sweet potato is a better choice in terms of your nutritional needs. And of course the RDAs are concerned with vitamins and minerals but ignore crucial analyses of fat, carbohydrate and protein content of foods. So, while a useful beginning, it's difficult to translate the RDAs into a healthy diet.

While nutritional labelling will be a great step forward for consumers, it will be of limited value. Though in 1975 in the USA it was believed that roughly 85 per cent of all manufacturers would be using nutritional labelling soon, by 1985 less than half of packaged foods in the USA were labelled. In the UK this figure was even lower. Moreover, some labels are almost deceptive. For example, a manufacturer must list ingredients in descending order of amounts. But sugar can be listed in various forms such as sugar, dextrose, corn syrup, honey, molasses, etc. If you're not experienced in reading labels, you can end up buying a product that has far more sugar than a cursory glance would reveal.

And while the labels might list the amounts of certain nutrients, this information still doesn't tell you what you need to know – which is: how much is good? If you know the amount of fat or protein or fibre or complex carbohydrates in a certain food, can you tell if it's a good choice in terms of the ideal, or in terms of what you've already eaten today? Most people just don't know if a food with 10 per cent complex carbohydrates is a good choice. And, finally, it is enormously time-consuming to stand in a supermarket and compare labels to check varying percentages of nutrients.

Nutritional labelling is good as far as it goes, but it doesn't give us any help with the foods we should be eating the most of: whole, unprocessed foods. You can check a label to see if Coco Pops cereal has more sugar than Fruit and Fibre, but there are no handy labels to help you determine whether a white versus a sweet potato, or an apple versus a banana, or a pork chop versus a veal chop, is a better choice in terms of your nutritional needs.

The fact is, nutritional labelling and the RDAs are a useful beginning, but for most people they are simply raw data in a form too complicated to be of much use. It's good to know that a product contains 15 per cent of your daily requirement of protein, but where do you go from there? Is that an acceptable amount? Is it a good contribution to your daily protein intake? And how does it compare to other similar products?

It's almost as if food labelling, which is of course a major stride forward in the interests of good nutrition, is only an intriguing set of puzzle pieces which the average consumer is unable to put together in any useful way.

Unfortunately, despite the enormous interest in nutrition today, the experts can't be of much help in determining which foods offer better nutritional value. They know that a bran muffin is better than a confectionery bar . . . probably . . . unless, come to think of it, the bran muffin is commercially manufactured with saturated fat and has lots of cholesterol . . .

No doctor or nutritionist can tell you which foods are best to eat because, up to now, they haven't had the 'software'. While the government has charts that list all the nutrient values in thousands of foods, they're not widely available and, even if they were, most people (including doctors and nutritionists) would be overwhelmed by trying to translate the vast sea of data into any useful information. It's just too complicated. The best anyone could do up to now was to point out that some foods are better than others. Some foods low in cholesterol are high in sugar or salt. Some foods low in calories have virtually no nutritive value. Some foods that are high in protein are surprisingly high in fat. Did you know that tofu, that favourite 'healthy' soya substitute for animal protein in many diet and vegetarian meals, is high in fat?

Nutripoints has made use of the most up-to-date information available on foods today. It's looked at nutritional labelling, the RDAs, calorie and cholesterol counts, etc. as *raw data* – which is what it really is as far as the consumer is concerned – and gone one step beyond this to provide the first accurate, practical nutrition guidebook.

How Diets Have Shortchanged Us
or Putting the Nutrients Back in Nutrition

Many people in the Western world are suffering from the first stages of malnutrition. How could this have happened? In large part, it's due to our obsession with dieting, which translates into a never-ending desire to lose weight. In fact, losing weight has become such a primary focus for so many of us that we forget that a 'diet' refers to a system for nourishing the body rather than a means to lose weight. When was the last time a friend told you he or she was on a 'diet' geared to improve their consumption of all the major nutrients so they could feel better and prevent disease?

In fact, many diets today take into consideration the negative elements in Western eating patterns and help you avoid excess fats, cholesterol and sodium – though very few help you avoid all three. And most diets make you feel as if you're the naughty child in primary school: the basic theme is 'don't, don't, don't; no, no, no'! Don't eat this; don't eat that; don't even think about eating all these things!

Nutripoints goes beyond this negative approach and moves the whole idea of diet into another, positive, realm. Most diets set you up for failure; there is no way you can 'fail' with Nutripoints. That's because the emphasis is not on avoiding certain foods, or only eating specific foods. Rather, the emphasis is on *choice*. The Nutripoint system assumes that you are intelligent and that you are ready to improve your diet. It provides you with the information – the kind of information you've never had before – that will enable you to make intelligent choices.

Most of us think of nutrition in terms of 'dieting' or losing weight. We think if we eat foods that are low in calories and avoid junk food, we're doing well. Unfortunately this focus on calories has obscured the crucial importance of adequate nutrition. The simple fact is that most of us are not very well nourished. We eat too much fat, too much protein, too much sugar and we don't get enough fibre, complex carbohydrates and certain crucial nutrients in our diets.

While Americans have reduced their fat intake 12 per cent since 1977 and slightly increased their complex carbohydrate intake, the British diet has not changed as quickly. While we're eating more yogurt than we were and more wholesome snacks (including fruits and nuts), our consumption of salty chips rose. We all claim we're eating fewer sweets, but consumption of 'gourmet' biscuits and cakes has increased. Who's eating all this stuff?

I witnessed a typical example of how some of our misguided notions about foods have more to do with trends than accurate information on how foods affect our bodies. I was in the supermarket watching a young man – well dressed with his briefcase under his arm – who was filling his trolley. He carefully chose a bottled water, a low-calorie frozen dinner, a large bottle of diet soft drink and then a huge bag of M&M sweets!

While most people today are at least aware of shortcomings in their diet – or at least aware enough to insist that they're doing better (despite the facts that contradict them) – they're still vulnerable to disease from too much fat and too little fibre.

The more surprising results of recent USDA and FDA surveys are that our diets are deficient in vital minerals and vitamins. As the two top officials of the US Department of Agriculture's Human Nutrition Information Service reported, '50% or more (of the 38,000 people surveyed) had intakes below the USRDA for vitamin A, iron, calcium, magnesium, and vitamin B6; over 30% of the individuals failed to meet the 70% RDA levels for these nutrients. Zinc and folacin [folic acid] are also known to be short in many diets.' The report concluded: 'U.S. diets do not show up well . . . when either the RDA or the [USDA's] Daily Food Guide is used as a standard'. So while most of us feel fairly complacent about the nutrients we're getting from our diets, the facts tell a very different story.

And the very steps we take to reduce fat – like cutting out red meat and many dairy products – are further reducing our intake of these important nutrients.

Does it really matter if your intake of, say, iron, is low? Most of us tend to think that a deficiency of any given nutrient is only a remote possibility. People believe that their iron intake must be OK if they don't have anaemia. What most people don't appreciate is the subtle interplay of nutrients in our bodies: it doesn't take a diagnosed deficiency to make you feel tired, or make it hard for you to shake off a cold. Indeed, lack of sufficient iron in your diet will begin to sap your energy and lower your physical and mental productivity long before it turns into a full-blown deficiency.

Also many popular reducing diets are unsound, and sometimes we make them even worse by adapting them to our own taste or 'inventing' our own diets where we simply cut out foods we believe to be fattening. In many cases, we end up eating a shockingly inadequate diet that repeats one or two 'low-calorie' meals virtually every day.

As I mentioned before, even people who eat a relatively good diet will unknowingly cut out essential vitamins and minerals when they reduce the fat and cholesterol in their diets. Most people simply don't know how to substitute a 'good' food for a 'bad' one. They're not aware that the right diet can be a simple matter of intelligent substitution.

I think that the goal of *optimum nutrition* will replace concern with the calorie as we learn more about the crucial role these nutrients play in ensuring our well-being.

As Paul Saltman, trace element researcher at the University of California, San Diego, says, 'There is every reason to believe that millions would have more energy, and would perform at higher levels physically and mentally, if our diet were richer in certain minerals and trace metals.' Nutripoints is the best method available today to help you achieve that goal.

The Advantage of Natural Nutrition

'Why can't I just take a vitamin pill?' How many thousands of times have I heard this question? It's not surprising that people are confused on the issue of vitamin pills. The vitamin pill manufacturers spend veritable fortunes convincing us that a pill is a just as good, if not better, source of nutrition than food. And who wouldn't *want* to believe them. You don't have to shop frequently for pills. They don't take up much room. You don't have to wash or chop or stir-fry or sauté them. But the fact is that vitamin pills have virtually no real role in achieving natural nutrition.

Did you know, for example, that most of these reports you hear about that demonstrate that Vitamin A or Vitamin C can cure or mitigate the effects of this or that disease *do not rely on pills but rather on food as a source of the vitamin*? Many people hear about research that promises to help their arthritis or pre-menstrual tension or whatever, and begin to dose themselves on whatever vitamin or mineral was cited as the cure. But frequently, pills had nothing to do with the reported results.

This is just one misconception about vitamins. As I'll demonstrate, there are other, even more compelling, reasons for relying on *natural nutrition* or fuel from food.

One of the cornerstones of the Nutripoints Programme is that *pills are not a substitute for food*. Here are some of the drawbacks of vitamin supplementation:

● *Even the best vitamins are incomplete.*

Despite what you may read or hear, vitamin supplementation is not an exact science. It's a relatively new scientific frontier: by 1913, only two vitamins had been recognized. Moreover, because we're interested in the effects of vitamins on humans and humans cannot be experimented with for obvious reasons, we're limited in how much we *can* learn about the effects of vitamins on human health.

But we do know a great deal from animal experimentation. For example, guinea pigs eating a totally synthetic diet that contains all the known nutrients needed to sustain their lives will not thrive. Why? Because we're not aware of all the essential nutrients – for guinea pigs or for man. Dr Jean Mayer, one of the most highly respected authorities on nutrition, has said that '. . . if the history of the development of our science is a dependable guide, there may be nutrients performing significant duties for us that we have not yet identified. In particular, there may be minerals functioning heroically to our benefit and all unknown to us'. A vitamin pill contains the *known* micro-nutrients and it's the best we can do. But no one can claim that it's complete.

Vitamin D2, or irradiated ergosterol, for example, can be produced by irradiating yeast with ultraviolet light. Because this is a 'natural' process, irradiated ergosterol can be called a 'natural' vitamin (in the USA). Milk and some other food products, as well as vitamin supplements, contain irradiated ergosterol. But this substance, Vitamin D2, is not the same as the D vitamin produced in the body when ultraviolet light strikes the skin. Moreover, Vitamin D2 does not supply the complex of D vitamins found in such foods as fish oils, milk fats from animals feeding on fresh greens, and liver. The simple fact is that the supplements we create, either 'naturally' or otherwise, may not be exactly the same as those created by nature in foods. If the effects of these created supplements in the body are precisely the same, no one can prove it, and there's room for great scepticism on the part of the consumer.

● *Even the best vitamin supplements are not perfectly balanced; some are dangerously unbalanced.*

The vitamins and minerals that occur naturally in food are balanced. Nature dictates how much of a given nutrient will be present. But the contents of a vitamin pill are dictated by companies –

companies that are run for profit, and that sometimes pander to the public's ignorance about vitamins and how they work in the body.

It's important to remember that nutrients have to work in concert and to take too much of one or another can be useless, or possibly even dangerous. For example, a slight increase of zinc may decrease copper retention as well as interfere with calcium absorption. Large doses of folic acid can mask a Vitamin B12 deficiency and result in serious and irreversible neurological damage. In pregnant women, large doses of folic acid can cause zinc deficiencies, which could lead to birth defects. Most people are astonished to learn that megadoses of Vitamin C impair Vitamin B12 utilization and can raise blood cholesterol.

Vitamins and minerals work in concert with one another and we ignore this fact to our peril. Calcium, for example, is one of the most abundant minerals in the body. It's found in bone, cartilage, teeth, blood and nerve cells. We're all conscious today about calcium deficiencies because of the threat of osteoporosis. But calcium supplements can do more harm than good. Calcium is used by the body in conjunction with magnesium. The body also requires Vitamin D for calcium absorption. One of these minerals taken alone will have a totally different effect. For example, magnesium oxide is effective in the relief of constipation. If you take it with calcium it will have no effect on your bowels. Excessive calcium stored in the body can result in a disorder called 'hypercalcaemia'. Calcium, taken in its natural form in dairy products and vegetables, is the only guarantee that the body is getting the calcium in concert with magnesium in the effective balance for optimal functioning.

The only way to be sure that the nutrients you ingest are properly balanced and readily absorbed by the body is to get them from food.

- *Vitamins can be toxic.*

The body stores excess Vitamin A in the liver. The fact that the liver is a storehouse for many excess vitamins is why it is also considered a valuable food (though liver has great drawbacks in nutritional terms which I'll go into later). In any case, the liver could almost be seen as one of the original megavitamins. And, like commercially produced megavitamins, it can be dangerous. For example, long ago Eskimos learned to avoid eating polar-bear liver. They knew it caused death;

although they didn't know that it did so because of its extremely high content of Vitamin A.

In the early 1960s, approximately twenty children in New York died from Vitamin A overdoses when their mothers doubled the recommended dosage of vitamin supplements. Each child took two capsules daily. And this was in addition to the already generous amounts of Vitamin A that the children were receiving from foods in their diets.

There are also long-term dangers to the use of supplements. For example, some experts worry that consumption of large amounts of iron supplements could cause a build-up of iron in the liver, leading to serious problems in later life.

● *Vitamin supplementation can alter your body chemistry.*

There's a more subtle problem relative to vitamin/mineral supplementation. While consumers may be aware that high levels of certain nutrients can be dangerous, most are not aware that even low routine doses of vitamins can create problems by conditioning the body to *expect* higher than normal levels of certain vitamins. This is known as 'systemic conditioning'. It occurs with water-soluble vitamins and it can create withdrawal problems when the nutrient is withdrawn. There is a great deal yet to be learned about systemic conditioning in relation to nutrients, but we do know that it can affect offspring as well as the individual taking the nutrient. There have been cases of infants suffering from something described as 'rebound scurvy', which causes temporary scurvy-like withdrawal symptoms because their mothers took megadoses of Vitamin C while pregnant. You should certainly never take megadoses of any vitamin while pregnant, without first consulting your doctor. If you are currently taking megadoses of a water-soluble vitamin (including the B vitamins and Vitamin C), be sure to cut down on your intake gradually to avoid the symptoms of withdrawal. (Megadoses of a fat-soluble vitamin should be ceased immediately if at toxic levels.)

You should also be aware that vitamin/mineral supplementation may alter the results of various diagnostic tests, particularly blood and urine tests. Large doses of Vitamin C can give false readings on blood in the stool and sugar in the urine. If you take supplements,

particularly in high doses, be sure to tell your doctor so that diagnostic tests can be correctly interpreted.

How to Take a Vitamin

Despite what I've just said, I'm not totally opposed to intelligent
vitamin supplementation. If you follow Nutripoints, there is really no
need for supplements. But some people just can't shake the belief that
a vitamin will give extra insurance. To these people I recommend a
single, balanced multivitamin taken *every other day or a half a*
vitamin taken daily. Even a person on a poor diet gets 50–75 per cent
of the RDAs and there's no need to supplement beyond this. There are
some groups who may benefit from a vitamin/mineral supplement:
young children, especially those who follow a special diet for
medical or cultural reasons; elderly people who eat a limited number
of foods; people on diets that contain fewer than 1,200 calories a day;
pregnant women; strict vegetarians who eat no dairy produce or eggs,
and people with certain illnesses that seriously impair the absorption
of nutrients. If you are on the lowest-calories version of Nutripoints,
you might also benefit from the half-a-vitamin-daily regime.

Here are some do's and don't's on taking vitamins

- Do take only a vitamin that offers close to, *but no more*
  than, 100 per cent of the RDAs for all nutrients. If the
  levels are a *bit* higher, they're not dangerous – but
  they're a waste. If they're a *lot* higher – some vitamins
  contain 1000 per cent of the RDA for one vitamin and 20
  per cent of another – they're really unbalanced and
  should be avoided.
- Don't go for the highest-price vitamin. Claims that
  vitamins are 'natural' as opposed to 'synthetic' really
  have no bearing on their effectiveness. And a national
  brand name may be no better than a much cheaper
  store's own brand.
- Do check the expiry date on any vitamins you buy. They

will become ineffective over time and are best used when fresh. Store them in a cool, dark, dry place.

- Don't waste money on vitamins that contain substances for which there is no proven nutritional need. Lecithin or 'Vitamin' B15 are two examples of such substances. Inclusion of the following in supplements only raises the price without any nutritional benefit: arsenic, cadmium, carnitine, choline, cobalt, lecithin, nickel, PABA, silicon, tin and vanadium.

- Unless you're under a doctor's orders, don't take vitamins that contain substances that are otherwise useless or dangerous. Fluoride, iodine and phosphorus are readily available elsewhere, in water, salt and protein foods respectively. Chloride, potassium and sodium are easily obtained from the diet. Molybdenum isn't a recommended mineral in supplements because risk of toxicity outweighs that of a possible deficiency. Moreover, even moderate amounts of molybdenum can cause a copper deficiency.

- Do take your vitamins with a well-balanced meal. Though there is evidence that *some* minerals are best absorbed on an empty stomach, most vitamins seem to be best absorbed when taken with foods.

Is Our Food Really Safe?

There is great concern today about the quality of our foods. The various additives and pesticides used to promote growth and storage life of foods are a troubling fact of life.

I have not taken into consideration additive and pesticide use in my Nutripoint scores for various foods for a number of reasons. First, most uses of pesticides and various additives simply don't make enough of a difference in the *nutritive* value of a food. Secondly, it is simply too difficult to calibrate. Apples, for example, come from so many regions and growers with so many varying methods of cultivation that it would be impossible to assess in a book such as this.

While Nutripoints cannot be your guide on how to avoid pesticides and chemicals in your food, I think it's important to be an aware and educated consumer. In 1989 there was a scare concerning the use of the chemical alar on apples. Many people stopped buying apples and apple products. But within a few weeks a number of supermarkets had released information regarding their apple supply so while some people were complaining about the limited number of juices they could safely give to their children others knew that there were at least a dozen apple juice brands that were perfectly safe. The lesson is be aware!

An excellent book that can help you make sense of the dangers of additives and pesticides is *E for Additives* by Maurice Hanssen (published by Thorsons, revised edition, 1987).

From a practical standpoint, how can you minimize the risk you take in eating certain foods? Here are some tips:

- Wash all fresh fruit and vegetables, and rinse them thoroughly.
- If the foods have been waxed, peeling is more effective than washing.
- Try to buy produce that originates within the EC. Other foods may contain residues of pesticides banned by the EC. You'll have to have the co-operation of your super-market manager to learn the source of produce in your market; sometimes, though, it may be hard to get this information.
- When possible, buy organically grown fruits and vege-tables or those grown under alternative methods of growing and cultivation to keep chemical use at a minimum.
- Request that your supermarket carry organically grown foods. Write to their headquarters and express your concern about pesticide residues.
- Write to the National Consumer Council about your concerns regarding pesticide use or, alternatively, the Department of the Environment or the Ministry of Agriculture, Fisheries and Food.
- To avoid the risk of salmonella, wash your hands thoroughly before handling poultry and eggs. Refriger-

ate raw and cooked poultry and eggs. Keep raw poultry and eggs away from cooked poultry and eggs. Cook eggs and poultry thoroughly. Wash surfaces that come in contact with raw poultry and eggs with warm soapy water.

For those who are concerned about contracting listeriosis, it is wise to choose pâté, cheese, etc. that have been pasteurized. In addition, since listeria is a widely distributed organism care should be taken to handle food hygienically and to reheat chilled foods thoroughly.

- To avoid parasites, don't eat raw seafood. Farm-raised fish and shellfish are much safer to eat raw than fish harvested in the wild.

Is Our Food Really Nutritious?

Many people today are concerned about the actual nutritional value of foods. In fact, many of my patients have mentioned that they take vitamins, at least in part, because they don't believe that the foods they eat, even supposedly highly nutritious foods, provide high-quality nutrients. They think this happens because of the use of fertilizers and the length of time foods must travel and spend on the supermarket shelves before we eat them.

Fertilizers used in commercially produced foods are not necessarily a negative in terms of good nutrition. It sometimes amuses me, by the way, that the same people who are opposed to using chemical fertilizers are often devoted to vitamin/mineral supplements, which are, after all, nothing more than chemical fertilizers for the body. That aside, you should not be categorically opposed to fertilizers or chemicals, as some of them actually preserve the nutrients in foods.

And what about the notion that foods are lacking in nutrients because they're grown in depleted soils? The fact is, the final agricultural 'product' – whether an apple, potato, carrot, or a beetroot – is primarily determined by that plant's genes, not the quality of the soil in which it grew. While the mineral content of a given food is partly determined by the soil in which it grew, you can rest assured that if a vegetable reaches the shops and it looks and cooks and tastes like a turnip, it's going to have all the nutrients that are normally assigned to a turnip.

Beyond pesticides and depleted soil, the question of storage in relation to nutrient contents is a valid one. But you might be surprised to learn that the greatest loss occurs in your own kitchen. When the analyses of various foods are done to determine their nutritional content, they're not done on rare, perfect, organically grown superfoods: they're done on the very same foods that you find on supermarket shelves. So when you learn that a raw red pepper has 140 mg of Vitamin C, you can be confident that the red peppers you buy in your supermarket have very close to the same amount.

Once the food reaches your kitchen, nutrition can be quickly lost through poor storage and processing. Most meats, fish, fruits and vegetables should be stored promptly in the refrigerator. They should be carefully wrapped. And they should be washed just before eating or cooking.

PART 3

The Nutripoint
Building Blocks

The Nutripoint Formula

When I was growing up, it was a meat and potatoes world. Children were supposed to drink their milk and eat their green vegetables and parents weren't supposed to eat too many calories. And that was just about the extent of common nutritional wisdom. But in my family there was someone who had a different view of the world, particularly the world of food.

My grandmother was one of the original 'health nuts'. At least, that's how some people viewed her when she arrived at our house with her health and nutrition magazines and her brewer's yeast. But I thought Grandma was someone very special. And, on the face of things, if what she was doing was 'nutty', at least it worked: she was full of energy and spirit and had one of the most positive approaches to life I've ever seen. She inspired me to believe that there was something to this idea of paying attention to what you ate. As she mixed up her 'breakfast concoction', I would be at her side, saying: 'Is this good for you?' 'Is that good for you?' 'Is this better than that?' 'How much better is this than that?'

Now I understand how I used to drive her mad: she really didn't have any way to answer me. And when patients began to ask me the same questions I often thought of her with a smile. I was in the same position as Grandma. I knew that some foods were bad, others good, but I didn't know much beyond that. The difference, though, was that Grandma was a grandma and I was a *nutritionist!* That inability to answer nutritional questions, a predicament seemingly handed down from one generation to another, was the original inspiration for Nutripoints.

As I worked with patients and struggled with their questions, I began to think how marvellous it would be if you could reduce nutritional information to simple numbers: just give each food a certain number of points for the good things it had. The major problem faced by my patients was the juggling act they had with all the nutritional variables. They had to think about cholesterol, sodium, total fat, saturated fat, sugar, complex carbohydrates, vitamins, minerals, fibre, caffeine and alcohol, in addition to calories. As one patient told me, 'I'd have to be a walking computer to work all this out.' I knew what he meant, because he'd need to refer to labels, and food composition tables and RDAs for his group of the population.

So in 1981 I worked out a rough formula. I tested it out on a computer using USDA (United States Department of Agriculture) data on 400 foods. It seemed to work and I was delighted, but I put it aside to focus on other things. Then when I came to the Aerobics Center in Dallas, I revived my old idea and began to use it with patients. I assigned numbers to foods to help people choose the best ones.

The idea of a food having a number attached was a big success and the patients loved it. But there was something missing. I needed a *system* – some method of helping people get a variety and a balance of foods as well as the best foods.

In 1985 I started using the basic concepts that evolved into Nutripoints: high-nutrient density; low calories; and balance. All this was done with numbers, and it was wonderfully effective. The patients at the Aerobics Center had serious health problems such as coronary heart disease, high cholesterol, high blood pressure, obesity and diabetes, and poor eating habits which were a major risk factor for all these diseases. While at the Center, they had great success with my 'numbers' system. There was just one problem with the early versions of Nutripoints. Patients used the numbers when they were at the Center but, once they got home and tried to find their way without the numbers, they had difficulty in sticking to their new, good eating habits.

I knew that if I wanted to help people stay with an optimum-eating programme, I'd have to come up with a complete system that not only rated the foods, but also allowed people to achieve variety and balance, *within the system*. And, of course, it had to be easy – no more complicated than the simple numbers I was already working with. My patients were intelligent professionals, and if *they* had such difficulty choosing the right foods and sticking to good eating habits, I could only imagine the problems that the average person who had never been exposed to a 'wellness clinic' must be experiencing.

I began to perfect Nutripoints, working with patients as I did so, to test its effectiveness and confirm its accessibility. It took countless hours with the computer and with data from food manufacturers and chains to come up with a programme that was, first of all, accurate – more accurate than anything currently available – in rating as many foods as possible. It had to make it easy for people to get a completely balanced diet, and I wanted them to be able to do it by picking their own favourite foods – or at least foods they liked – so the system had to be very flexible. And finally, it had to be easy. It had to be something that someone could do at home by themselves and something they could stick to whether they ate at home, at restaurants or at friends' houses. I'm finally satisfied that Nutripoints fulfils all these goals.

Here's how the Nutripoints formula is set up

First, I determined the components of each food: how much of each vitamin and mineral, fibre, protein, complex carbohydrates, cholesterol, total fat, saturated fat, sugar, caffeine and alcohol was in each food entry. There were eighteen *essential* elements and eight *excessive* elements in each food, the amount of which needed to be determined.

Where did the information come from? I used various sources. The Cooper Clinic Database provided about half the information. The USDA Database was enormously helpful. I also referred to Penn and Church's comprehensive book, *Nutritive Value of Foods*, as well as other nutrition books. In the case of brand name and fast foods, the information came either from the manufacturer's research data or from food labels. I wrote to approximately 150 companies and received information from more than three-quarters of them. In the cases of the fast foods, I wrote to manufacturers and included those foods that I received data on.*

Once I had gathered the information on all the foods, I needed to analyse it in terms of what nutrients the foods had and how they compared with how much of those nutrients we need in our diets. For

* The Nutripoint values appearing in the UK edition are based on data published by the Ministry of Agriculture, Fisheries & Food, and provided by food manufacturers and consultants.

example, a food that has a full day's requirement of Vitamin C is better than a food that has 50 per cent of a day's requirement of Vitamin C. So the nutrient content needed to be compared with a standard.

I wanted to use a standard for each nutrient that represented the highest level of *essential* nutrients per calorie, and also the lowest level of *excessive* nutrients per calorie. In that way, I'd be able to downgrade foods that are high in nutrients but also high in calories, or, say, a food that's very high in a mineral like calcium but also very high in fat. It's also an attempt to introduce a balance factor which limits credit for a single nutrient. If a food has 50 per cent of the USRDA for six nutrients, it's a better food than one that has 150 per cent of the USRDA for a single nutrient. And, by the way, a food can only get 100 per cent credit for an essential (even if it has 200 per cent of the RDA for a given factor), but there's no limit on how negatively the excessives can affect the Nutripoint score.

For my standard for the *essential* nutrients, I used the USRDA requirements for adults. United Kingdom RDAs are also provided here.

Nutrient name	USRDA requirement	UKRDA requirement*
Protein (high quality)	45 g ⎫	54–84 g
Protein (low quality)	65 g ⎭	(see note in text)
Vitamin A	5,000 IU	4,500 IU
Vitamin C	60 mg	30 mg
Thiamin or Vitamin B1	1.5 mg	0.9–1.3 mg
Riboflavin or Vitamin B2	1.7 mg	1.3–1.6 mg
Niacin	20 mg	15–18 mg
Calcium	1,000 mg	500 mg
Iron	18 mg	10–12 mg
Vitamin B6	2 mg	—
Folic acid	0.4 mg (400 mcg)	300 mcg
Vitamin B12	6 mcg	—
Phosphorus	1,000 mg	—
Magnesium	400 mg	—
Zinc	15 mg	—
Pantothenic acid	10 mg	—

* Source: DHSS, 1979.

The levels set by the US government are generally the highest standard for each nutrient based on the National Research Council's recommended daily allowance for different sub-groups of the US population. Therefore, these standards should meet or exceed the needs of virtually all healthy adults. As to the two kinds of protein, because we're rating each food individually we quantified the *type* of protein and the ratings reflect this. High-quality protein is found in animal products and low-quality protein is found in all other foods, and they're so defined because the balance of amino acids is more complete in animal protein. (In the UK, however, this split is not recognized.) But, in practice, you don't need to worry about types of protein because the balance of the Nutripoints Programme takes care of this for you.

The following essentials have no USRDA and therefore the following guidelines were used:

	US	UK*
Complex carbohydrates	60 per cent of total calories	—
Total carbohydrates	—	60 per cent of total calories
Dietary fibre	35 g†	30 g
Potassium‡	5,625 mg	—

* *Source: NACNE* (National Advisory Council on Nutrition Education), 1983.
† This is the upper limit of the daily recommendation of the National Cancer Institute in the USA.
‡ Although no USRDA for potassium has been set, the National Research Council has set a 'recommended safe dietary intake' of several nutrients including potassium. This level represents the highest level within that range.

The standards shown in the table on p. 54 were used as the upper limit allowable for each of the *excessive* elements in our diet. Once I set these standards, the computer converted these figures to a percentage of either the recommended amount (in the case of the essential nutrients) which would be a positive percentage, or the recommended limit (in the case of the excessive nutrients), which would be a negative percentage.

For example, an apple has 6 mg of Vitamin C. So I would take 6 and

	US	UK
Total fat	30 per cent of total calories	Same
Saturated fat	10 per cent of total calories	Same
Cholesterol	300 mg per day	—
Sodium	3,000 mg per day	3 g less/day
Sugar	10 per cent of total calories	Less
Caffeine	200 mg per day	—
Alcohol	½ oz of pure alcohol per day	Not more than 4 per cent of energy intake

divide by the USRDA for Vitamin C, which is 60. The resulting figure is 10 per cent. So for one of the 18 variables, Vitamin C, an apple scores 10 per cent. The Nutripoint formula does that calculation for each of the 18 essentials, adds all those percentages together, and then divides by 18 to come up with an average percentage of the RDA for each food.

Another example: an orange has 66 mg of Vitamin C, so 66 divided by 60 (the USRDA for Vitamin C) equals 110 per cent. An orange has 110 per cent of the USRDA for Vitamin C. But the formula gives no credit beyond 100 per cent for any one of the excessives. That's done to avoid giving too much credit to a food that is high in only one nutrient. We don't want a food to be at the top of the list if it has an enormous amount of one nutrient but not much of any other nutrient. So the percentage score for the orange in relation to Vitamin C is 100 per cent.

A variation of the same procedure is done for the excessives. For example, whole milk has 20 mg of cholesterol for an 8-oz (200-g) serving. Three hundred is the daily limit of cholesterol, so you determine what percentage of your daily limit is contained in that 8-oz glass of milk. Three hundred divided by 30 equals 10 per cent. Because it's a negative factor, this means it's a negative percentage. So milk gets a 10 per cent negative for cholesterol.

All of those percentages, negative and positive, for each food were then added together and divided by 18 – the number of factors. That percentage is then divided by the total calories in the standard serving of that food. The result is a fraction. The fraction is then multiplied by 1,000 and rounded to the nearest half or whole number.

The resulting figure is the Nutripoint rating for that food.

I ultimately considered 26 factors for each of the 1,500 foods in the UK Nutripoint system, which translates into 39,000 pieces of information that went into the rankings.

One of the advantages of the Nutripoint formula is that it's flexible. If another nutrient is discovered or another negative factor that affects our health is revealed, the formula can be adjusted for this new information and the numbers re-calculated to come up with new, updated Nutripoint scores for every food. It's a formula that's poised to adapt to the latest nutritional research, so that the Nutripoint score for a food will always be the best and most complete evaluation possible.

A Few Questions About the Nutripoint Formula

While I have just described the basics of how the Nutripoint formula works, there are some questions that commonly arise:

● *Are all the factors weighted equally?*

In other words, does a food get as much credit for having 100 per cent of the RDA of Vitamin C as it does for having 100 per cent of the RDA for pantothenic acid? And, is having too much fat just as bad as having too much caffeine? It becomes obvious when you ask these questions that some factors should be weighted, and this I did. The following are exceptions to the formula rules:

The following factor is weighted two times positive:
dietary fibre

I felt that fibre is of utmost importance in the Western diet, so I weighted it more positively to help steer people to foods that are rich in fibre. Weighting fibre highly also helps to lower the scores of foods that are fortified, because many of the latter have lots of vitamins and minerals but are low in fibre due to processing.

The following factors are weighted three times negatively:

cholesterol

alcohol

I felt that cholesterol was an extremely negative factor in today's diet. By weighting it with a triple negative I ensured that foods high in cholesterol would have lowered Nutripoint scores.

Because alcohol is negative in so many ways, I weighted it particularly negatively. It can be high in calories. It's virtually devoid of nutrients. It drains the body's stores of nutrients, particularly the B vitamins. It's a toxin. And it can be psychologically harmful. For these reasons, I wanted to steer people away from alcohol.

- *Could the formula for Nutripoints ever change?*

Yes. It's possible that we'd find a more accurate way to calculate Nutripoints, especially if there's a research breakthrough on a new nutrient or on an element that's revealed to be particularly harmful to our health. It's good to remember, however, that whatever flaws might exist in the system now, at least it is consistent in its analysis and is the best and most up-to-date analysis we have. Because it does the same things to all foods and because the foods themselves will not change, it's an extraordinarily reliable guide to food value.

- *How did you decide what the portion size should be for each food?*

The Nutripoint score is a *quality* rating. The serving size correlates with the calories in the food. In other words, the quality of the food times the calories equals Nutripoints. In order to make sure the Nutripoint value is correct, I had to be sure that the calories per serving within each group were approximately the same. I also had to be practical about amounts that people regularly consider to be a serving. Here's how the calories per serving break down in the various Nutrigroups:

Nutrigroup	Calories per serving
vegetables	20–60
fruits	50–100
grains	100–200

pulses/nuts/seeds	100–200
milk/dairy	100–200
meat/poultry/fish	125–250

and in the non-food groups:

oil	50–100
sugar	100–200
condiments	0–20
alcohol	100–200

The serving sizes get smaller as the amounts of calories and fats go up. If something has, say, 100 calories, you might have an 8 oz (200 g) serving, but if it's 200 calories, you might have a 4 oz (100 g) serving.

- Were there any surprises in the results of the Nutripoint food ratings?

Yes. For example, I was surprised at how low peanut butter rates. At 0.5 Nutripoints it's low down on the pulses/nuts/seeds Nutrigroup list. I thought that because it has no cholesterol and a considerable amount of protein, it would do better. I was also surprised at the cheeses. The fat and cholesterol in cheese really pulls it down and many types of cheese are below the recommended level in the milk/dairy Nutrigroup. This makes it obvious that it's important to stick to the low-fat dairy foods. I was surprised at how bad eggs are. While egg whites are fine, a whole hard-boiled egg is − 11.5: a terrible rating! It's really the cholesterol that pulls it down. Lean beef was also a surprise: it's not as bad as many people think. In fact, as you glance down the list you'll find that it's sometimes a better choice than some types of chicken. I'm sure you'll be interested to check your favourite foods in the lists and discover how they rate. You may be in for some surprises, too!

The Essentials and the Excessives

Now that you know the basics of what went into the Nutripoint formula, you might find it interesting to learn a bit more about the components of foods and how they affect your diet and you.

I have a slightly revolutionary proposition to make: let's look at the essentials of our diet in a completely new light. Instead of breaking things down into 'sources of energy' or 'percentages of daily requirements', let's be completely practical about what we need to know about food.

In fact, you don't *really* need to know anything but the numbers and groups of Nutripoints, but you probably have a healthy curiosity about the basic factors that go into working out the Nutripoint numbers. So let's look at food with a fresh approach.

The factors that have been worked into the Nutripoints formula are all elements in the foods we eat. Some are good for us and are lacking in our diets; others are good for us, but are consumed in excessive quantities; still others are bad for us and should be avoided. I've made a totally practical breakdown of the elements of foods that corresponds only to what you need to know. I've divided them into two groups: the essentials and the excessives.

My breakdown of the essential elements in our diet is slightly unconventional. The fact is that both fat and cholesterol, for example, are indeed essential to maintain life. But, because they have become problem elements in our diets, I've moved them into the 'excessives' category: no one in this country has to worry about getting enough fat or cholesterol in their diets. And calories, too, earn their place on the 'excessives' list, even though we couldn't live without them.

So my breakdown is as follows:

Essentials
complex carbohydrates
protein
dietary fibre
vitamins*
minerals†

* vitamins include A, thiamin, B2, B3 (niacin), B6, B12, C, pantothenic acid, folic acid.

† minerals include calcium, iron, magnesium, phosphorus, potassium, zinc.

Excessives

calories	sodium
total fat	sugar
saturated fat	caffeine
cholesterol	alcohol

The Essentials

There follows a brief description of the role of each of these elements in our diets.

Complex carbohydrates

Carbohydrates, as the name implies, are made up of carbon, hydrogen and oxygen. Carbohydrates supply energy in the form of blood sugar to keep the body functioning. Carbohydrates have always seemed to me to be a 'schizophrenic' food group: on the one hand, complex carbohydrates – those found in cereals, rice, breads, pasta, beans, nuts and all vegetables – are really good for you. You probably eat too little of them, and one of the efforts of Nutripoints is to ensure that you eat more. On the other hand, simple carbohydrates – those found in refined sugars like sweets, cakes, puddings, soft drinks, sugar-coated cereals, etc. – are terribly bad for you, and you probably eat too much of them. Nutripoints has separated out sugar as a negative factor in the Nutripoint formula and complex carbohydrates as a positive factor, so the numbers reflect what you really need in your diet. In other words, Nutripoints weights fibre as a positive factor and sugar as a negative factor; the system highlights the best carbohydrates for you.

The Nutripoints Programme emphasizes complex carbohydrates as a primary food. By recommending 10 servings of carbohydrates daily (4 of vegetables, 3 of fruits, 2 of grains and 1 of pulses/nuts/seeds), it recognizes that a diet rich in complex carbohydrates can improve your energy levels and your performance, as well as help you prevent long-term disease. This emphasis on carbohydrates has replaced the old-fashioned reliance on protein as a 'diet' food. Carbohydrates are low in fat, but none the less very satisfying. They are rich in vitamins and minerals. They 'burn clean' in the body, leaving only carbon dioxide and water to be excreted. (As opposed to protein, which leaves potentially dangerous nitrogen and sulphur waste.) Carbohydrates are also the major source of fuel to the brain, which relies on an optimum level of blood sugar to function properly.

Protein

Along with fat and carbohydrates, protein is one of the sources of energy from food. It is essential for life. Every cell in the body contains some protein. Indeed, excluding water, half of the body's weight is protein. It's important that you get sufficient protein in your diet every day to function at an optimum level.

Most of us think of protein as the 'safest' food component. We think carbohydrates are bad; we *know* fat is bad. But protein is something that you should eat a lot of, especially if you're on a diet. Right? Wrong! Most of us eat at least *twice* as much protein as we need. And, unlike a water-soluble vitamin, excess protein is not excreted. It's stored in the body. Since the major sources of protein that we consume include meat and dairy products, which are high in fat, our high protein intake is also creating high fat, cholesterol and calorie intakes. In short, it's making us fat. Not only is excess protein making us fat, it's also putting a strain on the liver and kidneys, which are responsible for processing the excess protein. Finally, excess protein consumption increases your need for calcium, and can exacerbate problems connected with a low-calcium diet.

The Nutripoints balance assures you that you're getting just the right amount of protein daily. You'll be getting high-quality protein with a balance of all the essential amino acids. But the source of some of your protein will shift: instead of getting most of your protein from meat, you'll be getting more from other sources such as pulses. I might mention here that I've provided a Vegetarian Option, which is a Nutripoints programme for those readers who prefer to omit meat entirely from their diets.

Top tip: protein. The best approach to giving your diet a better balance in terms of protein is to shift the major source of it from meat and dairy foods to fish, soya products (like tofu), and dried beans and peas. There are some excellent main course frozen dishes that rely on tofu as the main source of protein. They're low in calories, without cholesterol, and low in fat. I highly recommend them.

Fibre

Fibre, commonly called 'roughage', is a non-nutritive part of food. It has virtually no calories and is not digested. Fibre is important in giving 'bulk' to food and helping to move it through the intestines and colon. Lack of sufficient fibre in the diet has been linked to cancers of the colon and rectum, diverticulitis, haemorrhoids, hiatus hernia, varicose veins and heart disease.

There are two kinds of fibre present in foods: soluble and insoluble. We've long been aware of insoluble fibre. It was the 'rough stuff' that we could depend on to promote regularity. It's insoluble because it won't dissolve in hot water. Soluble fibre, which will dissolve in hot water, has an effect on the body's metabolism of fats and sugar. Oat bran has become the most popular soluble fibre – maybe because we can put it into sweet, fatty muffins and think we're doing ourselves a nutritional favour! While it's certainly true that certain soluble fibres have a beneficial effect on blood cholesterol, fruit and vegetables, as well as beans, contain soluble fibre that's every bit as beneficial as the fibre found in oat bran.

Following the Nutripoints Programme will ensure that you're getting enough of both soluble and insoluble fibre. There is no need to take fibre supplements: they can actually be dangerous if you don't take them with enough water, or if you take them to excess. Moreover, too much fibre, which is more likely to occur if you take supplements, can rob your body of important nutrients as it moves food too rapidly through your digestive system. Remember: food, not pills!

Regarding the oat-bran craze, which has recently been superseded by the rice-bran craze, it seems that every few months there's a new nutritional bandwagon you can climb on. It may be megavitamins or fibre or tryptophan or fish oil. As appealing as these trends can be – it's always so tempting to think that you can change and improve your life in one easy step – most of us who have seen these trends come and go recognize that they're often an exaggeration of some very complex research. The oat-bran phenomenon started with some research that found that the fibre in certain foods, including beans, carrots and oat bran, among others, was helpful in controlling cholesterol. Well, carrots and beans are not new so everyone seized on the oat-bran connection. In fact, oat bran is no more effective in controlling cholesterol than a number of other fibrous foods. But who wants to eat beans or carrots when you can have a huge, rich, sweet, fatty oat-bran muffin for breakfast and feel virtuous at the same time? The fact is, if you're serious about good nutrition, the trends are not your best inspiration. So often they turn out to be exaggerated or even wrong.

Nutripoints is beyond trends, in that you'll be eating the very foods that may be discovered in the near future to be 'wonderfoods'. How can I be sure of this? Because you'll be eating the very best, highest-quality foods. Nutripoints makes optimal nutrition an achievable goal today.

Top tip: fibre. Beans are an excellent source of fibre and play too small a role in our diets. To get the most benefit from beans, soak them overnight and then cook them slowly at a low temperature. If you don't soak them but then cook them in boiling water, you'll just toughen them and impede the availability of the fibre and nutrients they're rich in. (Note: kidney beans must be boiled fast for at least 10 minutes.)

Vitamins and minerals

Adequate vitamin and mineral intake is one of the major goals of Nutripoints, and the system ensures that you'll receive more than adequate amounts of every essential vitamin and mineral.

Vitamins are organic substances that are essential to biochemical reactions in our bodies. Vitamins do not give us 'energy'; we rely on calories for that. They simply promote the metabolic functions that result in energy. There are 13 vitamins. Four vitamins are fat-soluble (A, D, E, and K) and nine are water-soluble (C, and the eight B-complex vitamins, including thiamin, riboflavin, niacin, B6, folic acid, B12, pantothenic acid and biotin).

Minerals are inorganic substances that, like vitamins, promote various metabolic functions in the body. The macrominerals, which are needed in relatively large amounts, include calcium, phosphorus, magnesium, potassium, sulphur, sodium and chlorine. The microminerals, or trace minerals, are needed in tiny amounts. They include iron, zinc, selenium, manganese, molybdenum, copper, iodine, chromium and fluorine. I haven't included the microminerals in the Nutripoint formula, because they're not normally reported in nutritional data and getting information on amounts available in foods is difficult if not impossible. It's also been shown that foods high in the macronutrients are also high in the micronutrients.

Here's a quick breakdown of every vitamin and mineral considered in the Nutripoint numbers, and some tips on how to guarantee your intake of that particular substance.

VITAMIN A

I think of Vitamin A as the 'wrapper' vitamin, because it's largely responsible for the health of our wrappers: our skin, hair, and mucous membranes (including the linings of our mouths, stomachs, etc.). It's also involved in vision, immunity and reproduction. Vitamin A is fat-soluble. The most exciting news about Vitamin A is that researchers have recently connected a lack of Vitamin A with the development of certain cancers. This is important news because many of us, particularly children and adolescents, don't get nearly enough Vitamin A. At the same time, there is fear among medical experts that some people, hearing of the ability of Vitamin A to boost the immune system and prevent cancer, are overdosing on this vitamin. Because Vitamin A is fat-soluble and is therefore stored in the body, toxic amounts can build up and cause jaundice or liver damage. The good news is that, because the body stores Vitamin A – it can store a year's supply – you don't have to worry about maintaining an extremely high daily consumption. And if you're getting your Vitamin A from foods (where it occurs in the form of beta carotene), you never have to worry about the dangers of overdosing.

Top Tip: vitamin A. One of the best, quickest and most delicious sources of Vitamin A is a sweet potato – it gives you twice the RDA for Vitamin A. If you've never tried a baked sweet potato, you're missing something. Just eat them hot from the microwave plain, or with a bit of virtually fat-free yogurt for a delicious snack or as part of a meal.

VITAMIN C

Vitamin C, or ascorbic acid, is one of the best-known water-soluble vitamins. It's a sort of 'glue' vitamin that is important in the manufacture of the collagen that helps hold the body together. Perhaps one of the best-known roles of Vitamin C is that of infection fighter.

I've learned that many people, even those who don't take any other kind of vitamin, will take a Vitamin C tablet regularly or when they feel a cold coming on. This obsession is somewhat misguided, as most of us get at least one and a half times the amount of Vitamin C we need each day. But at least Vitamin C, because it is water-soluble, is not one of those vitamins that can readily become dangerous in high levels: the body excretes excess amounts.

Top Tip: vitamin C. I think the best Vitamin C 'supplement' you can take is sweet, red pepper. One-eighth of a red pepper – or just a few strips – will give you about 95 mg of Vitamin C, or one and a half times your daily requirement. And red pepper is very low in calories.

VITAMIN B1 (THIAMIN)

Vitamin B1 is known as the 'energy' vitamin, because one of its most important roles is in the metabolism of carbohydrates. It's also important in the functioning of the nerves. It stimulates growth and good muscle tone, and it has also been shown to stabilize the appetite. Because thiamin is water-soluble, it's rarely dangerous – even when taken to excess.

Top Tip: vitamin B1. Don't add baking soda to water when you cook vegetables (as some people used to to retain bright green colours). This practice depletes thiamin (as well as Vitamin C). Don't boil rice in lots of water and then drain it. Instead, measure the appropriate amount of rice and the appropriate amount of water (about twice as much water as rice) and then cook till all the water is absorbed. Throwing out water that rice has boiled in is like throwing out 'vitamin soup'.

VITAMIN B2 (RIBOFLAVIN)

Vitamin B2 is necessary for carbohydrate, fat and protein metabolism. It boosts the immune system and the formation of red blood cells. It also promotes good vision and helps keep skin, nails and hair healthy.

Top Tip: vitamin B2. Rely on dairy foods! Because so many of the sources of Vitamin B2 are foods low in Nutripoints, like offal (which are very high in fats), low- or non-fat dairy foods are your best source. Keep up with the Nutripoint food groups, and don't neglect your two servings of high-Nutripoint dairy foods daily. Adding some extra non-fat dried milk when you're baking, or to recipes like meat loaf, can give you a good boost of Vitamin B2.

VITAMIN B3 (NIACIN)

Vitamin B3 has become a 'hot' vitamin these days because of the role it plays in reducing cholesterol. In addition to this crucial job, niacin is necessary for carbohydrate, fat and protein metabolism. It helps maintain the health of your skin, tongue, digestive system and nervous system.

The good news about niacin is that very few people have problems with deficiencies, because the vitamin is so readily available from so many food sources. Just 3 oz (75 g) of water-packed tuna, for example, supplies about three-quarters of your daily requirement.

Because of reasons discussed in the chapter on vitamins and their dangers, I don't recommend that you try to supplement with niacin to lower your blood cholesterol unless you're doing so under the direction of a physician. There are serious side-effects connected with megadoses of niacin.

Top Tip: vitamin B3. The highest level of the RDA for niacin (for males 19–22 years old) is 19 mg. As 3 oz (75 g) of tuna canned in water has 14 mg, you can see that niacin is not hard to come by in food. So my suggestion on niacin is to avoid supplements. Prolonged use of megadoses can result in skin rashes, irritation of peptic ulcers, irregular heartbeat, jaundice and promotion of gout among other symptoms.

VITAMIN B6 (PYRIDOXINE)

Vitamin B6 is a water-soluble vitamin that has many roles in the biochemical life of the body. It's necessary for fat, carbohydrate and protein metabolism. It's important in the production of red blood cells and of antibodies. It helps to regulate blood-glucose levels. Because Vitamin B6 is crucial to so many functions, its lack is signalled by a wide variety of symptoms – and has been connected to everything from asthma and pre-menstrual tension to diabetes, cancer and cardiovascular disease.

In the United States so many people are so deficient in Vitamin B6 that the US government has named it a 'problem nutrient'. Because B6 plays such a crucial role in so many biochemical activities in our bodies, it's important to get an adequate amount. But please don't rely on supplements. While B6 is water-soluble and excess amounts are largely flushed from the body, high doses (upwards of 200 mg a day) can result in nervousness, insomnia, frequent urination, irritability and wetting the bed in children.

Top Tip: vitamin B6. One banana will give you over a third of your daily requirement of Vitamin B6.

VITAMIN B12

Vitamin B12 is a water-soluble vitamin that is responsible for the formation of blood cells as well as the metabolism of carbohydrates, fats and proteins. It's important for cell replication and helps maintain a healthy nervous system.

Because Vitamin B12 is found in so many foods, it's rare to suffer a deficiency. The people most likely to suffer a B12 deficiency are vegans (vegetarians who do not eat *any* animal produce), and even they are not very likely to suffer a deficiency if they vary their diet.

Top Tip: vitamin B12. Stores of B12 can last in the body for up to fifteen years. As you only need 3 mg daily, you really don't need to worry about a deficiency and you can easily see why supplements of B12 would be superfluous for healthy people.

PANTOTHENIC ACID

Pantothenic acid (also known as Vitamin B5) is essential for healthy skin, body growth and the production of antibodies. It's also necessary for the conversion of fats and carbohydrates into energy. Because pantothenic acid is so readily available in foods, there's little danger of deficiency.

Top Tip: pantothenic acid. Because you need such small amounts and because it's so readily available, you'll have no trouble getting adequate pantothenic acid.

FOLIC ACID

Folic acid aids in the metabolism of proteins and is necessary for the growth and division of cells. Folic acid is essential to your mental and emotional health.

Folic acid deficiencies are rare but women may be more vulnerable. If you're taking contraceptive pills or if you've been taking aspirin because of its connection to mitigating the development of cardio-vascular disease, you may need extra folic acid in your diet. A number of health problems are related to folic acid deficiencies, including depression, infections, cervical dysplasia in women on the pill, and cancer.

The emphasis on vegetables and pulses in the Nutripoints Pro-gramme will guarantee that you'll receive an adequate supply of folic acid. Folic acid is readily available in green leafy vegetables – those that are at the top of the Nutripoints list are rich in the vitamin. Even if you're among those who need extra folic acid, you'll be more than adequately supplied by the Nutripoints Programme.

Top Tip: folic acid. To retain the most folic acid in your foods, cook vegetables in the least possible water – stir-frying them in the smallest possible amount of oil is a good method.

The best possible folic acid boost is a spinach salad: 4 oz (100 g) of raw spinach gives you twice the RDA of folic acid.

CALCIUM

Calcium is one of the most abundant minerals in the body, essential for human life. Calcium sustains the maintenance and development of bones and teeth, and is crucial for blood coagulation, muscle action, heartbeat, and nerve function.

Calcium has been in the news for a few years now and with good reason. Those especially vulnerable to calcium deficiency are women: adolescent girls and middle-aged women. The deficiency shows up in later years when these women suffer from osteoporosis – a weak bone structure that can lead to dowager's hump and easily fractured bones.

One of the reasons people have become at risk for calcium defi-ciency is that many of the foods that have high levels of calcium also have high levels of fat. Milk and dairy products, which are the most common sources of calcium, are often avoided by people on a low-fat diet.

Unfortunately, many people have resorted to calcium supplements to try and increase their calcium intake. Many people do this without even being aware of what their daily intake is in the first place, so they may be getting overdoses that could be potentially dangerous. Over-doses of calcium can result in kidney stones, constipation, and acid stomach, nausea or high blood-pressure complications. I strongly recommend that you avoid calcium supplements, and rely instead on the high-Nutripoint foods listed in the Milk and Dairy food group for the best low-fat sources of calcium.

Top Tip: calcium. 4 oz (100 g) of cooked broccoli or 4 oz (100 g) of low-fat yogurt will give you over a third of your daily requirement, while 4 oz (100 g) of cooked bok choy (Chinese cabbage) will give you well over a third. 2 oz (50 g) of non-fat dried milk gives you over a third of your daily requirement, and it can be added to foods like dressings, baked foods, meat loafs, etc. to boost calcium supplies without adding many calories.

IRON

A trace mineral essential for life, iron is the 'blood mineral'. It's necessary for the formation of haemoglobin, the red pigment in blood cells, which transports oxygen in the body. Iron deserves attention because it is so commonly deficient in the average diet. The National Food survey reveals that the iron intake of a large proportion of the UK population barely reaches the recommended level. Women are prone to iron-deficiency, particularly as a result of blood losses during menstruation.

Of all the nutrient-deficiency diseases, anaemia is the most common. And if you find it hard to translate a condition like anaemia into real-life problems, you'll be amazed to learn that one study of women found that their 'work performance' quadrupled when they increased their iron intake.

Top Tip: iron. You can dramatically increase your iron intake by taking some Vitamin C in the form of, say, orange juice with an iron-rich meal. Orange juice with breakfast, for example, can boost the absorbed iron by 200 per cent. Avoid drinking coffee or tea with meals: they decrease iron absorption.

MAGNESIUM

Magnesium is essential for every biological process. It aids in the body's use of carbohydrates, fats and proteins, and works in conjunction with other minerals including calcium, phosphorus and potassium. Many of us risk becoming deficient in magnesium because of **our low-calorie diets of highly processed foods.**

Top Tip: magnesium. 4 oz (100 g) of fresh, cooked spinach has about one-quarter of your daily magnesium requirement. Dried bran cereals like All-Bran, Bran Buds and Bran Flakes are good sources of magnesium, with 1 oz (25 g) of many of them providing about one-quarter of your daily requirement.

POTASSIUM

Potassium is the third most abundant element in the body. It works with magnesium to help regulate the heart, and with sodium to help regulate blood pressure and send nerve impulses. Fortunately, potassium is abundant in the average diet and so rarely poses the problem of deficiency. People who might be in danger of potassium deficiency include those suffering from a digestive disease, those using diuretics, and people with uncontrolled diabetes. Athletes and others who sweat profusely may find that their potassium levels are low.

Top Tip: potassium. If you are an athlete or if you exercise heavily in high temperatures, you should be wary of potassium depletion. Watch for weakness or fatigue over a longer than usual period of time. A quick recovery can be effected with a 'natural potassium supplement': a glass of orange juice or a banana. Avoid potassium supplements as overdoses pose serious risks.

PHOSPHORUS

You have a pound and a half of phosphorus in your body. Along with calcium, it's the most abundant mineral. Phosphorus, again along with calcium, is the bone mineral: it's responsible for the building of bones. It also plays a major role in other metabolic functions, including cell reproduction and conversion of foods to energy.

Because phosphorus is so widely available in a variety of foods – in dairy products, meats, fish, grains, nuts and beans – you rarely have to worry about a phosphorus deficiency.

Top Tip: phosphorus. If you frequently take antacids that contain aluminium, this can block your absorption of phosphorus. Check with a pharmacist to find an antacid that doesn't contain aluminium, or try to boost your phosphorus intake.

ZINC

Zinc is a crucial trace mineral that promotes growth and healing. It aids the immune system in its efforts to prevent disease and is important in a wide range of metabolic activities.

Marginal zinc deficiencies seem frequently to be the price paid for today's style of eating. Low-calorie diets are often the culprits as they sometimes provide only half the calories necessary for our daily zinc intake. Because of zinc's crucial role in boosting the immune system, this is a potentially dangerous nutritional situation. Zinc deficiencies also play a role in eating disorders such as anorexia nervosa and bulimia, osteoporosis, low sperm counts, gum disease, foetal complications including low birth weight, and other disorders.

Top Tip: zinc. One oz (25 g) of the following cereals will provide you with nearly a third of your daily zinc requirement: All-Bran, Bran Buds, Nutri-Grain, Special K; 3 oz (75 g) of lean pot roast will give you half your daily zinc requirement. And 3 oz (75 g) of raw oysters will give you 400 per cent of your daily zinc requirement!

The Excessives

The excessives are the elements in our diet that there are just too much of. As I mentioned before, most of these items are not totally bad; indeed, all of them, with the exception of caffeine and alcohol, are in fact essential to human life. It's just that our eating patterns have emphasized these elements to our detriment. We simply can't continue to eat diets high in fat, calories, cholesterol, sodium and sugar without paying the price in both long- and short-term symptoms and diseases.

Here are the excessives that have been worked into the Nutripoint formula:

total fat	sodium
saturated fat	sugar
calories	caffeine
cholesterol	alcohol

FAT

Fat has become one of the biggest problems in our diet. While fat is essential for life – as a concentrated energy source, a carrier of the fat-soluble vitamins, and a source of essential fatty acids – too much fat is ultimately life-threatening. And most of us are eating three to five times the amount of fat we need to keep our bodies functioning. We really only need the equivalent of one tablespoon of fat per day! All the excess fat we're eating is contributing to heart disease, colon and breast cancer, as well as obesity (which is linked to a number of other diseases).

Cutting down on fat is one of the single most important things you can do to improve your diet, and thereby extend your life. Nutripoints will make it easy for you, as fat is heavily weighted as a negative factor. By sticking to the foods that are at the high end of the Nutripoint food lists, and by being sure to limit your meat and dairy servings and portions to the Nutripoint recommendations, you'll be keeping your fat intake to 30 per cent of your total calories, and your saturated fat to within 10 per cent of your total calories – figures that are well within the limit set by the Committee on Medical Aspects of Food Policy. (We separate saturated fat from the total fat because, while foods with saturated fat don't necessarily contain cholesterol, they cause the body to produce cholesterol, and thereby raise serum cholesterol levels.)

Top Tip: fat. I think that the 'fat booby traps' are margarine and salad dressings. Many people avoid butter because it's high in saturated fat. Margarine is a better choice, but margarine is still essentially fat! You can't use it with abandon. Don't pile it on bread and sandwiches. You can eat a waffle with fresh fruit without missing the margarine at all. Get out of the 'fat spreading' habit. Salad dressings pose another danger, because many people find that they're eating more salads and vegetables on the Nutripoint Programme. But salad dressings are loaded with fat. Even if you do virtually no cooking, you owe it to yourself to find a good low-fat commercial dressing or make up your own using lemon juice or vinegar, or yogurt. You'll find such a dressing every bit as tasty as those oily ones, and far more healthy. Make up a batch and keep it handy in your refrigerator. You can even bring a small amount with you to a restaurant and ask for a salad without dressing, so you can add your own.

CALORIES

Hi-cal, low-cal, no-cal – calories have been the dominant issue in the way most of us have approached nutrition for the past thirty years.

All we want to know about calories is how to avoid them, and this obsession has given us a distorted picture of what nutrition is all about. Many books give endless lists of the calories in every imaginable food, and the premise of such books is that you can lose weight by substituting low-calorie foods for high-calorie ones; but, if you binge, as you no doubt will, you can catch up by eating next to nothing until you're back to your goal. This is all fairly basic, but the implication is that you can substitute, say, a bar of chocolate for a tuna sandwich made with wholemeal bread, and get away with it if the calories in the two foods are the same. I'm surprised that this old-fashioned approach to nutrition is still given any credence at all. The fact is that calories are just one of many factors that need to be considered in the decision as to whether a food is good or bad, nutritious or not.

Strictly speaking, calories are units of heat measurement: a calorie is the amount of energy it takes to raise the temperature of 1 g of water 1 degree centigrade. Calories are the fuel that enable our bodies to perform their endless metabolic tasks. The average adult man burns approximately 2,500 kilocalories per day and the average woman, 1,800 to 2,000. You need to consume about that many calories for your body to function: if you have less, you'll force your body to call on stored energy and you'll lose weight; if you have more, you'll store the excess calories as fat and gain weight. It's that simple.

Many of us are overweight. Some of us are overweight to the point where it seriously affects our health. Probably *most* of us believe we are overweight by at least five or ten pounds. Many of us think that if we could only restrict our caloric intake for a while, we'd get back down to what we weighed as students, or when at secondary school, or whatever our personal 'golden age' was. But most of us hate 'diets' because they're boring or hard to follow, or they make you feel sick or dizzy. In fact, I can promise you that you don't have to restrict the amount of food you eat. With the Nutripoints Programme you'll find that you can eat far more than you might have thought, but you'll lose or maintain your weight (depending on your goal) by eating foods that are more nutritious and lower in calories.

Top Tip: calories. I think the best thing you can do for yourself is to forget about calories. In the course of working with thousands of patients, I've found that the people who are the most knowledgeable about calories are also those with the most finely developed ability to 'cheat' on a diet. If you can recite the number of calories in a Mars Bar or Marathon, and think that if you skip a breakfast of equivalent calories it's OK, you're only fooling yourself! *Don't worry about calories; focus instead on Nutripoints.*

CHOLESTEROL

There is a 50 per cent chance that your blood cholesterol level is higher than 'desirable'. A significant number of people have a blood cholesterol level that is high enough to warrant medical attention.

Though controversy continues on the precise meaning and implications of blood cholesterol levels, there is no doubt that a high level puts your life in danger, and the tragedy of coronary heart disease – contributed to by high levels of blood cholesterol – is that for 40 per cent of its victims, the first warning sign is a fatal heart attack.

High levels of cholesterol have become the hidden time bombs in our post-war diet – a diet that's rich in fatty foods. We're now seeing the effects of a lifetime on such a diet: an increased risk of serious coronary heart disease which is now the number one killer in this country. High cholesterol levels are the major contributor to this epidemic. Indeed, among the people of the famous Framingham, Massachusetts, study, who have been tracked now for more than 40 years, only those with a cholesterol level below 150 mg/dl (3.9 mmol/l) have been found to be free of risk from premature death due to clogged arteries. Fortunately, the effects of a high-cholesterol diet can be mitigated.

You've no doubt been reading a great deal about cholesterol for the past few years, but you may also be confused about how to translate research reports into your own 'heart safe' diet. Nutripoints will eliminate this confusion because cholesterol is one of the major negative factors used in the Nutripoints Programme. The higher the cholesterol level of a food, the lower in Nutripoints.

On the Nutripoints Programme, cholesterol intake is limited to 300 mg daily, which is in keeping with the recommendations of the American Heart Association. In addition to simply limiting cholesterol intake, Nutripoints lowers serum cholesterol levels by emphasizing fibre and limiting saturated fat in the diet. This abundant fibre in the diet binds with bile acids which contain cholesterol, and thereby transports cholesterol out of the body.

The average person who follows the Programme will see a 14 per cent reduction in two weeks, depending on how high their cholesterol was to begin with. (If it's very high, the reduction tends to be greater; in our 'live-in' programmes at the Center, I've seen drops from 25 to 50 per cent in people with high cholesterol. It wouldn't be unusual for someone to go from 250 mg (6.5 mmol/l) to 180 mg (4.7 mmol/l) per 100 ml blood.)

If you are already suffering from coronary heart disease, the Nutripoints Programme is a safe and practical way to keep your cholesterol intake at the lowest possible levels. Simply stick to the food items near the top of the list, and avoid those below the recommended level.

Here's a breakdown I did that you might find interesting. It identifies the worst offenders in terms of *both* cholesterol and calories. These foods show a high ratio of cholesterol to calories and are thus double threats. Each entry has more than 1 mg cholesterol per calorie.

Food	Cholesterol per calorie (mg)
sweetbreads	10.2
lamb's kidney, fried	3.9
egg yolk	3.7
herring roe, soft, fried	2.9
egg, scrambled	2.8
egg, fried	2.7
omelette/ham & cheese	2.3
caviar	2.2
squid, boiled	2.1
paté, chicken liver, tinned	1.9
squid, raw	1.8
egg salad	1.7
shrimp/prawn steamed	1.7
mussels	1.5
spinach salad/egg, bacon, ham	1.5
beef heart	1.3
beef liver, fried	1.3
crab, tinned	1.2
sauce, cheese	1.0

Here are a few facts about cholesterol.

Cholesterol is a waxy substance found only in animals. Cholesterol in food is referred to as 'dietary cholesterol', while cholesterol in our bodies is called 'blood' or 'serum' cholesterol. Though both these substances are the same, they differ in origin: the body ingests cholesterol found in animal-based foods, and it also manufactures its own cholesterol *in response to consumed cholesterol*. While the body needs cholesterol to function, it doesn't need to *consume* any. The body is capable of manufacturing enough cholesterol to fulfil all its needs. The trouble with consuming large amounts of cholesterol is that it stimulates the body to overproduce cholesterol, and reduces its ability to remove dietary cholesterol from the bloodstream.

The ultimate result of excess cholesterol is clogged arteries, as the cholesterol adheres to the walls of the veins and impairs their ability to carry oxygen through the body. Among many other things, blood carries a regular supply of oxygen to the heart and, without oxygen, the heart muscle weakens causing chest pain, heart attacks and eventually death.

Here are five recommendations to help reduce your blood cholesterol levels:

1 Eat less high-fat food, especially those foods high in saturated fat.
2 Replace part of the saturated fat in your diet with unsaturated fat.
3 Eat less high-cholesterol food.
4 Choose foods high in complex carbohydrates.
5 If you are overweight, reduce your weight.

Nutripoints is a simple way to help you achieve all five of these goals.

By the way, you'll notice as you look at the food rating lists that some foods have a notation regarding cholesterol. This is because some foods like offal, while very high in nutrients, are also very high in cholesterol. If you are on a diet to lower your cholesterol, you should avoid such foods, even though they may be high in Nutripoints. There is a further explanation of this in the 'Notes' section just before the lists (see page 139).

Here is a complete breakdown of all the sources of cholesterol in your diet. When you see one of these listed on a food label, you know the food contains cholesterol, or is a vegetable product which doesn't contain cholesterol but is high in saturated fat which can raise your serum cholesterol levels. (Just 1 g of saturated fat is equal to eating 20 mg of cholesterol in its effect on your serum cholesterol levels!)

animal fat	hardened fat or oil*
bacon fat	hydrogenated vegetable oil*
beef fat	lamb fat
butter	lard
chicken fat	meat fat
cocoa butter*	palm kernel oil*
coconut*	palm oil*
coconut oil*	pork fat
cream	turkey fat
egg and egg-yolk solids	vegetable shortening*
ham fat	whole-milk solids

* sources of saturated fat

SODIUM

Sodium is a mineral that helps regulate blood pressure, and is essential for the proper functioning of the nervous system. Sodium is essential to life and, indeed, there are traces of sodium in almost everything we eat. There is more than enough sodium occurring naturally in foods to fulfil our daily requirements. The problem is that many of us consume 10–25 times the amount – about one-tenth of a teaspoonful – that we need.

Excess sodium can cause serious health problems, including high blood pressure which can lead to stroke, heart and kidney disease. A proportion of the population is genetically prone to developing high blood pressure by eating a diet that is too high in salt.

How do we avoid excess salt? Well, of course, Nutripoints has made it easy for you. Just choose foods from the top of the list and you'll be eating a diet that is naturally low in sodium. In addition, I recommend that you avoid processed foods whenever possible. The simple fact is that salt is added to so many processed foods in such large amounts that, if such foods are a mainstay of your diet, it's very difficult to avoid sodium. For example, a recent article reported the following surprising fact:

- 1 oz (25 g) of Kellogg's Corn Flakes has almost double the amount of sodium as 1 oz of Planters Cocktail Peanuts: 260 mg versus 132.

This demonstrates that if you need to restrict your sodium intake, you'll have to do more than simply shun table salt. For one thing, sodium by itself is tasteless; it's in the form of sodium chloride that it becomes the common table salt we think of. But sodium by itself is still added to foods. Fortunately, some manufacturers are now including labelling that will help you make low-sodium choices.

You should also be aware of other sodium-containing ingredients that could be listed on a package including monosodium glutamate, baking soda (also identified as sodium bicarbonate), garlic salt, brine and sodium citrate.

Because so many of my patients are concerned about sodium intake, I'm including a list of salt substitutes to use for added food flavour.

Sherry (avoid 'cooking sherry' as it's high in sodium)
lemon juice
lime juice
garlic powder
onion powder
vinegar (including balsamic, rice wine, apple, red wine, raspberry, and blueberry vinegar)
ginger
cumin
pepper
green chilli peppers

Top Tip: sodium. There are a number of ways to reduce the sodium in your diet – such as simply cutting out table salt, which you may well already be familiar with. But one that I always pass on to my patients is the following: if you rinse tinned tuna in brine with tap water for one minute you will remove 80 per cent of the sodium! This is an especially useful tip because tinned tuna without oil is so high in Nutripoints. It's also useful to rinse tinned vegetables before cooking.

SUGAR

Sugar, along with cellulose and starch, is a principal component of carbohydrates. The body does need glucose – one of the components of sugar – to function. But sugar, as opposed to starch or complex carbohydrates, is quickly digested – there's little or no fibre to slow the absorption of the sugar – and gives you an immediate burst of energy. Complex carbohydrates, on the other hand, are usually rich in fibre. They burn more slowly and give the body a more stable energy supply, as well as providing nutrients.

The drawback of sugar as a source of energy is that it contributes far too many calories in return for a very small contribution in terms of nutrients. This drawback would make sugar a nutritional waste, but it's also involved in other physical problems. There's no doubt, for example, that a high sugar consumption contributes to dental caries. There is also some evidence to link excess sugar with diabetes, heart disease and obesity. It's so dense in calories that it makes it very difficult for the average person to burn off all the calories they're consuming in a day when sugar is a major component of their diet.

Despite sugar's poor nutritional value, some of us get an amazing 20 per cent of our total daily calories from sugar. This means that we're eating 20 to 30 teaspoons of sugar *each day*! That's an incredible amount of sugar, and we just can't afford it either in terms of weight control or in terms of the nutrients we need each day. Even if you never add sugar to any food you eat, you're still overdosing on it if you don't know how to read food labels. Did you know, for example, that most of the calories in some ketchups and salad dressings come from sugar? Some of the mixes you use to coat meats with before roasting have a significant percentage of sugar. Everything from bacon to baked beans and soups, from gravy mixes to spaghetti sauces, can have large amounts of hidden sugar. And you probably know that some breakfast cereals have enormous amounts of sugar; indeed, a few cereals have so much sugar that it's actually the main ingredient. (And they'll still run advertisements claiming to be 'part of a balanced breakfast'!)

Sugar is by far the most popular food additive. But if you learn its various disguises, you can avoid it. Here are the various forms of sugar you'll find listed on food labels:

brown sugar	caramel
corn syrup	dextrin
dextrose	fructose
glucose	grape sugar
honey	invert sugar
lactose	maltose
maple sugar	molasses
sorghum syrup	

If you see any of these ingredients listed among the first few on a label, you know the product is high in sugar. Sometimes manufacturers will add sugar in a variety of forms. For example, you'll see corn syrup, dextrin and molasses all listed in various places in the label. Even if they're not among the first ingredients, you can be sure that the product has plenty of sugar; it's just that the sugar is composed of a few different types, but if you added them all together, it might well be the first or second ingredient.

Of course, you don't really have to worry about reading labels, because Nutripoints has done the work for you. The numbers have accounted for the amount of sugar in foods.

One final word about artificial sweeteners. Patients always ask how I feel about them. The primary artificial sweetener that I sanction is NutraSweet.* It's the only artificial sweetener that's a natural substance. It's a protein that is actually metabolized and used by the body. Saccharine is not a nutritive substance, and because it must be excreted by the body, it has a potential – when taken in excessive amounts – to cause cancer. Unlike NutraSweet, however, saccharine is heat-stable, and can be used in cooked products.

On the other hand, because NutraSweet is a natural substance in an *unnatural* form (it has been processed), there may be some potential problem with it that has yet to be discovered. I therefore recommend

* Phenylketonurics should be aware that NutraSweet contains phenylalanine, and individuals with this condition should avoid this.

that you limit yourself to two drinks and one food product sweetened with NutraSweet per day.

As to the question concerning NutraSweet's effect on blood sugar, I wondered if it might have an indirect effect on raising blood sugar. I used myself as a guinea pig and here's what happened. While in a fasting state, I drank 12 oz of Diet Pepsi (sweetened with NutraSweet) and then tested myself on a glucose meter. The Pepsi had no effect on my blood sugar. An hour later, I drank a glass of cranberry juice (which is very high in sugar) and the meter shot right up – thus showing an elevated blood sugar. Obviously, this isn't a scientific study, but it allayed my own fears as to the effect of NutraSweet on my blood sugar.

Top Tip: sugar. Satisfy your sweet tooth nature's way with fruits that are naturally sweet. Water melon is a good choice. And frozen grapes, while not particularly high in Nutripoints, can make a great snack – freezing them makes them last longer!

CAFFEINE

Caffeine is a stimulant that blocks the effects of our brain's natural tranquillizing agent, allowing the brain to move temporarily into a higher gear. It affects blood pressure and heart rate and increases respiration. It's a diuretic as well as a vasoconstrictor and vasodilator: it allows the blood vessels of the brain to constrict and those of the heart to dilate.

Caffeine's positive effects are undeniable: it gives a boost of energy and temporarily sharpens mental acuity; it also allows you to concentrate on monotonous tasks.

But caffeine is a drug. The dangers of caffeine addiction are real. Though links between caffeine and heart disease and cancer have largely been disproven, there remains a real connection between caffeine consumption, digestive diseases and anxiety. It's the more subtle effects of caffeine that are troublesome to most of us, often because we never make the link between caffeine consumption and our minor symptoms. If you suffer from insomnia, afternoon fatigue, tension headaches and general anxiety, you might be suffering from the effects of caffeine addiction.

I suggest that you have no more than two caffeinated drinks per day. I recommend that you stick to decaffeinated soft drinks and decaffeinated coffee and tea.

Top Tip: caffeine. I think freeze-dried decaffeinated coffee or grain-based drinks such as Caro Extra or Barley Cup make good substitute drinks. Just be careful that you don't lighten your coffee substitutes with cream! Use skimmed milk, or try it black.

ALCOHOL

Alcohol is both a toxin and a drug. It's a toxin because the liver must work to detoxify it. That's why you always hear of liver damage among alcoholics; the liver is simply exhausted from its labours to detoxify a constant intake of alcohol. Alcohol is also a carbohydrate, though it's almost an 'anti-nutrient' because it increases your need for other nutrients while contributing almost nothing of any nutritional value of its own. Alcohol is also a drug that acts as a sedative. It anaesthetizes the brain beginning with the frontal lobe, or reasoning section, and moving on to the speech and vision centres.

Most of us have a schizophrenic view of alcohol: we accept and perhaps even enjoy its regular use for ourselves and among friends, but we deplore the countless lives it can ruin when abused. The problem, of course, with alcohol is control, and there can be a fine line between 'regular' and 'addictive' consumption of alcohol.

In addition to the seriously dangerous properties of alcohol, many people don't realize that alcohol can be destructive of nutrients. It will deplete stores of, or limit the body's absorption of, such nutrients as calcium, riboflavin, folic acid, iron, zinc, thiamin, and Vitamins B12, C, D and A. What this means is that if you regularly consume alcohol with meals – say a glass of wine with lunch and dinner – you may be counteracting the benefits of many of the nutrients you're consuming in those meals.

I think the healthiest alternative is not to drink at all. But, if you wish to drink, then you should take the 'damage control' approach: I suggest you limit yourself to one or two drinks daily. Avoid the spirits that are at the bottom of the Nutripoints Alcohol list, and stay with wines, wine coolers, beer and low-alcohol beer.

Top Tip: alcohol. Why not try some of the alcohol-free beers or lagers? Some of the brands have an excellent flavour, and can help break a bad habit if you're accustomed to, for example, having a beer when you get home from work. I also suggest that you try some of the mixed drinks *without* alcohol – a Virgin Mary is a good choice as it's spicy and has lots of flavour.

PART 4

Nutripoints at Work

This section of the book is devoted to everything you need to know to use the Nutripoints Programme in your daily life. It will answer all your questions from 'Can I get *too many* Nutripoints?' to 'What foods on a Chinese restaurant menu are the best choices?'

First, a simple breakdown of how to make the most of Nutripoints:

- *If you only used Nutripoints to help you choose one food over another*, for example as a guide to selecting a vegetable with a higher score (spinach at 53.5 Nutripoints instead of a baked potato at 8.5 Nutripoints or a chicken salad sandwich (wholemeal bread) at 4.0 Nutripoints rather than a ham and cheese sandwich (wholemeal bread) at 0.5 Nutripoints), you would improve your diet. But you would not ensure that you get all the essential vitamins and minerals, or that you get optimal amounts of protein, carbohydrates and fibre. And it will not ensure that you avoid excess calories, cholesterol, total fat, saturated fat, sodium, sugar, alcohol and caffeine.
- *If you only used Nutripoints to choose one food over another and tried to get 100 Nutripoints per day from a variety of foods*, you would upgrade your diet and get a sufficient amount of every vitamin and mineral. But you would not get optimal amounts of protein, carbohydrates and fibre. And you would not be avoiding excess calories, total fat, saturated fat, cholesterol, sodium, sugar, alcohol and caffeine.
- *To get the full benefit of Nutripoints, you must select foods that will give you a daily score of at least 100 Nutripoints, while staying within the serving limit for each group and meeting the minimum required servings for each Nutrigroup.* This is the most complete and effective use of Nutripoints. This use of the system will

ensure that you get 100 per cent of all necessary vitamins and minerals; that you get optimal amounts of protein, carbohydrates and fibre; that you avoid excess calories, cholesterol, total fat, saturated fat, sodium, sugar, alcohol and caffeine.

Your Current Nutripoint Status

Before you begin using the Nutripoints Programme, I recommend that you take stock of your current eating habits. The best way to do this is by keeping a food diary for three days. The most immediate benefit of making a three-day food diary is that it will allow you to analyse your current diet in terms of Nutripoints. It will instantly pinpoint the weaknesses in your diet. It will give you a powerful incentive to get started on Nutripoints, and it will also serve as encouragement when you begin to see how quickly your diet improves and your scores go up with just a few basic changes in your eating habits.

Keeping a food diary is also a helpful way to get used to using Nutripoints in your daily life: you'll become familiar with the Nutrigroups and get to know the highly rated foods.

Keeping a Food Diary

When patients come to the Cooper Clinic, I always ask them to make a record of what they've been eating for three typical days. You have an advantage over these patients: you can make more accurate records because you'll be doing it as it happens. (You'd be amazed at how much some of us can eat, almost unconsciously. If you tried to recall *everything* that you ate two days ago, could you?)

Accuracy really counts, so please don't try and fool yourself. Remember that you don't have to show these lists to anyone if you don't want to.

I suggest that you buy a new notebook, just for your Nutripoint scores. You might abandon it after a while, but in the beginning you'll find it very helpful. You need to jot down exactly *what* you ate and in *what amounts* for each meal. It's best to record *typical* days; they don't have to be consecutive. In other words, you can record a Wednesday (skip Thursday because you were travelling and not eating typically), a Friday and Saturday. It's a good idea to include one weekend day as well as two weekdays. Don't forget to record snacks, beverages, and condiments. Try to make your notes as soon as possible after a meal or snack, so you can remember whether it was three or five biscuits you had.

Try to record your portion sizes as accurately as you can. Typical portion sizes would be 8 fl oz (225 cl), 1 teaspoon, 1 tablespoon, 4 oz (100 g), 2 slices, etc.

Here's a table that will help you judge portion sizes:

Typical portion sizes

Meat, poultry, fish
3 oz (75 g) = size of palm of woman's hand (don't count fingers!)
= amount in a sandwich
= amount in a ¼ lb hamburger (cooked)
= chicken breast (3 in across)
6 oz (150 g) = restaurant chicken breast (6 in across)
= usual luncheon or cafeteria portion
8 oz (200 g) = usual evening restaurant portion

Cheese
1 oz (25 g) = 1 slice on sandwich or hamburger
= 1 in cube or 1 wedge aeroplane serving
4 oz (100 g) = 1 scoop cottage cheese

Salads
side salad = dinner salad
main-meal salad = salad bar salad

Potato
1 small = 2½ in long
1 med. = 4 in long
1 large = 5 in long (restaurant portion)
1 huge = 6 in long (meal-in-one potato)

Vegetables
2 tbsp = cafeteria or restaurant portion
= coleslaw or beans at a restaurant

Fats
1 tsp (5 g) margarine/butter = 1 pat
3 tsp = 1 tbsp
1 tbsp mayonnaise = typical amount in sandwich
2 tbsp dressing = typical amount on a dinner salad
= 1 small ladle (restaurant)
= ½ large ladle (restaurant)

Beverages
1 fl oz (25 ml) = 1 measure of alcoholic drink
4 fl oz (100 ml) = typical juice portion
= small glass of wine
8 fl oz (225 ml) = common milk portion
12 fl oz (325 ml) = 1 can of beer or soft drink

Here's a typical part of a daily record:

Meal	Food	Serving size
dinner	chicken breast (baked, no sauce)	4 oz (100 g)
	baked potato with	1 medium
	margarine	2 pats
	cheese sauce	2 fl oz (4 tbsp)
	cauliflower; steamed	4 oz (100 g)
	apple; fresh	1 large
	dinner roll; no margarine	1 small
	semi-skimmed milk	8 fl oz (225 ml)
snack	popcorn	1 oz (25 g)
	Coke	12 fl oz (325 ml)
	chocolate bar with nuts	2 oz (50 g approx) bar

After you have the three-day list, check each food portion with the Nutripoint values in this book. The easiest way to do this is to use the Alphabetical Lists at the back of the book.

You're going to want to know three things for each of your food diary entries:

1 portion size
2 Nutripoints
3 Nutrigroup

A sample 'Nutripoint Daily Record Sheet' is shown on page 89 to help you work out how to list your foods so that you can readily see how you're doing on points and portion sizes.

You'll want to check each food you consumed to learn how many Nutripoints your serving had. The alphabetical listing will probably contain any food that you might have eaten. Check it for each of the entries in your food diary. Be sure to check the portion size listed. If you ate 8 oz (200 g) of something and the Nutripoints are calculated at 4 oz (100 g), you must double your Nutripoints. Conversely, if you ate 4 oz (100 g) of something and the Nutripoints are calculated at 8 oz, you have to halve your Nutripoints for the particular food. If you can't find a precise food listed, work out the components of that food

Nutripoint daily record sheet

DAY:

Food Selection	Portion size	Veg.	Fruit	Grain	Pulses	Meat	Milk	Other	
					NUTRIPOINTS				
Breakfast:									
Lunch:									
Dinner:									
Totals									
Goals		55	15	10	5	5	10	0	100

and make an estimate. For example, if you had a salad that was composed of rice and mayonnaise and some chopped vegetables, check the values of each of these ingredients and add them up to arrive at a Nutripoint score for that food.

In addition to checking your daily Nutripoint scores, you want to determine the balance of your diet and whether you're getting the necessary variety. So when you check the Nutripoint score for each food, also check each food's Nutrigroup – e.g. meat/fish, grain, vegetable, etc.

Remember that the daily Nutripoint goal is 100 points divided among the six Nutrigroups as follows:

The daily Nutripoint recommendations

Servings	Nutrigroups	Nutripoints
4	vegetables	55
3	fruits	15
2	grains	10
1	pulses	5
2	milk/dairy	10
1	meat/fish	5
	Total	100

Now it's time to analyse your scores. Here are the three factors you're looking at:

1 How many of the six Nutrigroups do you have points in? This will give you an idea of how varied your diet is.
2 Did you achieve the recommended number of servings for each Nutrigroup? This will show you how well balanced your diet is.
3 Did you achieve your Nutripoint goal of 100 points for the day? This will show you how nutritionally sound your diet is.

Here's a little chart that suggests a simplified way to analyse your daily score. You just fill in the Nutripoints for each of the required servings of each Nutrigroup. You can then readily see if you've reached your goal for that Nutrigroup and for the day. You may well find that when you make up your food diary, your scores and/or servings are way out, but this chart will at least give you a very visual way of analysing your numbers.

Nutrigroup	Servings	Nutripoints	Goal
Vegetables		=	55
Fruits		=	15
Grains		=	10
Pulses		=	5
Milk/dairy		=	10
Meat/poultry/fish		=	5
Your total:			100

From the countless surveys I've done on the diet histories of patients, I've learned that there are certain patterns in the average diet. Most people find that their biggest weakness is that they don't get nearly enough variety and balance in their diets. Indeed, most people seem to get nearly all their foods from only three out of the six Nutrigroups: meat/poultry/fish; milk/dairy; and grains. Some people fare even worse and omit grains as well. Most people get few, if any, pulses. And many people are short on fruits and vegetables.

Many people have what I think of as 'miscellaneous' diets: they get lots of meat and dairy foods along with lots of miscellaneous items that don't fall into any Nutrigroup – such as sugar, fat and condiments.

The average person gets 50 to 100 Nutripoints daily *even when eating considerably more than the allotted number of servings.* This means that the average person is getting a poor nutritional bargain in their daily diet: less – sometimes *far* less than required – at a cost of more calories than they need.

By using the system, then, you can get 100 to 200 Nutripoints daily in *significantly* fewer calories, thus enjoying a more nutrient-dense diet. And you can usually achieve this without making noticeable cuts in the *amounts* of food you eat.

Upgrading Your Diet

It's time to refocus your approach to food with the help of Nutripoints. Unless your diet is truly terrible, I think you'll find this an easy shift to make. Many patients tell me that they're delighted to find that, rather than being an 'authoritative' diet plan that urges you to eat tons of lettuce or grapefruit or some other food you might not like, Nutripoints leaves the choice up to you!

Your food diary has revealed where your diet is weak. You're probably not eating enough different kinds of foods. Most people find that just by paying attention to balancing their diet, they improve it enormously. So you'll probably need to work on getting sufficient servings from the various Nutrigroups. But how do you choose foods *within* each group?

Step 1: First I suggest you do your own personal food survey. Go through the lists by Nutrigroups and check the foods that you eat regularly. Are they high in Nutripoints? If so, great. If not, it's time to think about eliminating the foods that are low in Nutripoints, or at least those that are below the recommended level for each Nutrigroup.

Step 2: Make a list of the foods that you like and eat regularly that are high in Nutripoints. This will be the basis of your new, upgraded diet. These are the foods you can rely on because you already know that you like them and that they are high in Nutripoints.

Step 3: Now you need to focus on *variety*. Go through the lists by Nutrigroups again and look for foods that you like, or like but rarely eat. Make sure that you don't neglect the Nutrigroups you're weak on. (You'll know from your food diary if, for example, you rarely eat vegetables or fruits.) Perhaps you found that you *never* eat pulses. Well, now's the time to go through that Nutrigroup list and find some pulses that you like. Work out how you're going to work them into your diet. When you first begin with Nutripoints, you may find that it's difficult to work in two servings of pulses every day. This is perfectly OK. Many people have a sort of transitional stage where they substitute one meat serving for one of the pulse servings.

It's very important to remember that *variety* is as important as a high Nutripoint score. This pertains to choosing foods *within* a Nutrigroup as well as choosing foods *among* Nutrigroups. Remember that each food has its own unique 'fingerprint' of nutrients that identify it: it will be strong in some, weak in others. If you consistently pick only the top four, say, vegetables, you'll be missing out on the nutrients available in other vegetables that you need. Keep in mind that as long as you don't go below the recommended level of foods, it's better to have a variety within a list than an extremely high score.

Step 4: An excellent way to upgrade your diet is to use Nutripoints as the basis for making *substitutions* in your diet. You would do this between foods within a single Nutrigroup. For example, say you eat a lot of pork. You might want to scan the meat/poultry/fish Nutrigroup for a food with a higher Nutripoint level – fish, for example. Or perhaps you like spinach and lettuce equally: next time you make a salad, include lots of spinach and you'll be boosting your score.

Substitutions can be particularly useful when cooking. Here are some effective substitutions:

> Instead of butter use sunflower oil or low-fat spread.
> Instead of double cream use evaporated milk.
> Instead of full-fat cream cheese use a low-fat alternative.
> Instead of one whole egg use two egg whites.
> Instead of full-fat yogurt use sour cream, low-fat yogurt or virtually fat-free yogurt.
> Instead of sugar use NutraSweet.
> Instead of salt use a salt substitute.
> Instead of coffee or tea use decaffeinated, Barley Cup or herb teas.

Step 5: Another way to upgrade your diet is to use Nutripoints to alter your food choice. For example, say you eat a lot of fried chicken. Why not stick with chicken if you like it, but try grilling it instead of frying. Or make your beefburgers with a leaner grade of beef. Or, if you already eat grilled chicken, why not boost your score by taking the skin off before you grill it? If you love fruit, why not have some melon instead of your usual apple?

You can make these changes in each Nutrigroup. In the milk/dairy group you can change from full-fat cheese to low-fat cheese; from whole milk to semi-skimmed milk and then on to skimmed milk. You can go from 2 eggs to one whole egg plus one egg white.

Nutripoints makes it easy for you to upgrade your diet simply by familiarizing yourself with the lists. You simply look for a version of a food you like with a higher Nutripoints score.

How do you keep track of your Nutripoint scores through the day? You can continue with your food-diary notebook or you can use a sheet like the following, which not only will help you keep track of your scores, but will also make keeping track of your servings from the various Nutrigroups automatic. (This chart is for those who want to consume 1,000–1,200 calories per day; your chart can be personalized for your desired calorie intake, according to the guidelines on pages 99–102.)

Date		*Food*	*Nutripoints*
Breakfast:	1 grain		
	1 milk/dairy		
	1 fruit		
Lunch:	1 meat/pulse		
	2 vegetables		
	1 grain		
	1 fruit		
Dinner:	1 meat/pulse		
	2 vegetables		
	1 grain		
	1 milk/dairy		
	1 fruit		

Nutrigroup	*Servings*		*Nutripoints*	*Goal*
Vegetables		=		55
Fruits		=		15
Grains		=		10
Pulses		=		5
Milk/dairy		=		10
Meat/poultry/fish		=		5
Your total:				100

Obviously, you might want to alter this pattern on some days. Perhaps you'll have a fruit snack instead of a fruit dessert, or perhaps you'll have a grain as a snack instead of with dinner.

A Note on Water . . .

There is one nutritional 'essential' that I didn't include in the Nutripoint formula for obvious reasons: water. Your body is actually two-thirds water – forty to fifty quarts – and we can't forget that it's every bit as essential to life as food.

Most people don't give any thought to the amount of water they drink, but I think it's important to do so. You should be sure to drink six to eight 8-ounce (175 to 225 ml) glasses of water per day. Some people find it helpful to put six pennies in their right pocket in the morning and move one to their left pocket each time they drink a glass of water. It helps them keep track of what they're really consuming. Following the Nutripoint guidelines for your servings of these liquids, you can substitute diet soda or fruit juice for your water servings, but don't count caffeinated coffee or tea because they act as diuretics. If you exercise, of course, you should increase the amount of water.

Nutrigroup Trends

Many people have asked me what food types, in general, seem to be the best bets in terms of Nutripoints. It's interesting to point out that there are various trends in each Nutrigroup. If you're familiar with them, you'll be better able to choose high-Nutripoint foods, even if you don't have the charts at hand. I should mention again, by the way, that you can only compare Nutripoint ratings *within* each Nutrigroup. Each Nutrigroup has a nutrient 'fingerprint' with certain nutrients that it's high in, and others that it's low in. So, while you *can* compare apples and oranges, you *can't* compare apples and spinach.

Here, therefore, are some of the major trends in the Nutrigroups:

Vegetables: When you're looking for the top vegetables, think light and fluffy! Green leafy vegetables like turnip tops, spinach and watercress all have terrific scores. After the leafy vegetables, which you can readily see would be both low in calories and high in nutrients, we have the chunkier cruciferous vegetables like broccoli, cauliflower, asparagus, brussels sprouts, etc., which are very high in Vitamins A and C (the vitamins some doctors recommend you focus on as a step to reduce your cancer risks), as well as fibre and calcium. Next, in terms of scores, we have carrots and the more watery vegetables like okra, tomatoes, and potatoes, which are also high in Vitamins C and A as well as fibre.

All the top vegetables have a tremendous ratio of nutrients per calorie, but as you continue down the list you'll find that processing and the adding of salt and fat lower the scores of even an excellent vegetable. Keep in mind when choosing vegetables, that *all* vegetables above the recommended line (see p. 123) are very good foods, and there's no need to worry about sticking to the very top of the list for your four daily servings: as long as you are choosing from above the recommended line, you shouldn't have any trouble getting your 55 Nutripoints.

Fruit: The first trend we notice in the fruits is that the tropical fruits top the charts. Melons are right at the top along with papaya, guava, mango and kiwi. These fruits are packed with nutrients (including Vitamin C) and fibre, and extremely low in calories for their volume. After the tropical fruits we find the citrus fruits, including the orange, mandarin orange, tangerine and grapefruit. And then come the berries including raspberries, blackberries and cranberries. Most of the fruits are high in Vitamins A and C and fibre, with moderately high levels of other nutrients. Again, once we get below the recommended line, the addition of sugar, salt or fat lowers the scores. Foods like apple pie (at − 2 Nutripoints) gets about as far as you can from the basic nutritional appeal of the apple. And a cherry pie does even worse (at − 5 Nutripoints). Jams, jellies and preserves hit rock bottom, where virtually all nutrition including fibre has been processed out of the food and masses of sugar has been added. Robertson's strawberry jam (at − 5 Nutripoints) tells of the decline of the strawberry to the absolute bottom of the fruit chart.

Grains: At the top of the grains list you find the highly fortified cereals. There's some controversy about fortification but, in order to keep the system honest, I had to put the cereals where they fell. (Please note the caveat about fortification on page 139.) The very best cereals are those with the most balance in their fortification, as well as those that began with a good-quality natural food with plenty of fibre and complex carbohydrates. Kellogg's All Bran is at the top of the list. As we go down the line, we'll find cereals that are less balanced in terms of fortification, or cereals with less fibre or more sugar. The top rated natural (unfortified) cereal is wheat bran at 26.5 Nutripoints, followed by wheat germ at 10.5 Nutripoints, and Weetabix at 6.5 Nutripoints.

So a breakdown of the cereals shows that fortified whole grains top the list, followed by bran and then germ and then the other whole grains and then, as you begin processing and reducing the amount of whole grain and adding sugar, salt and fat, the scores decline. You'll find a terrible choice for breakfast is that 'health' food of the 1960s – granola – in the form of Granola Bars at − 2.0 Nutripoints.

As you move down the grain list, you find the various breads (topped by wholemeal bread at 6.0 Nutripoints), rices and pastas. Pizza makes a respectable showing, and gives an opportunity for those who must eat at fast-food restaurants to make a choice that will give them a grain serving that will make a positive contribution to their daily Nutripoint score. Pizza Hut's Pepperoni pan Pizza, for example, weighs in at 3.0 Nutripoints for half a piece. Any good cereal for breakfast that scores above 7.0 Nutripoints (and most do) followed by a Pizza Hut lunch would give you your two grain servings above your 10 required Nutripoints for that Nutrigroup for the day.

Pulses: Pulses are strangers to most people, though it's time you became familiar with them. They're a good protein alternative to meat; they're high in fibre; high in complex carbohydrates; low in fat and cholesterol; and high in nutrients. In our pulse Nutrigroup, we include not only peas and beans, but also nuts and seeds. Bean sprouts top the list at 18 Nutripoints, and it's easy to have them handy to put in sandwiches in place of lettuce, as well as adding them to salads. Sprouting increases the nutrients in the bean as it takes on nutrients in the water and develops a higher nutrition profile. Peas follow sprouted beans on the list. They're high in fibre, protein and complex carbohydrates, as are the next items on the list, mung beans. Down a bit from the beans is an excellent meat substitute – the frozen vegeburger which is made from soya. (By the way, these soya-based foods are processed foods, and can be difficult to digest. I therefore suggest that you use them occasionally as substitutes or convenience foods, but not as regular components of your diet.)

After the beans and peas and tofu come the nuts. They provide protein, but they're rated lower because they're high in fat (though of course it's not as saturated as the fat in meat). Remember, by the way, that there's no cholesterol in any vegetable product. As you descend on the list you find the adulterated foods which have been processed, and suffered the addition of salt and sugar. Even peanut butter makes a dismal showing, because of the addition of salt and sugar.

Milk/dairy: Since milk is an animal product, it's a good source of complete protein. It contains all the essential amino acids that the body can't produce. And, of course, it's high in calcium and complex carbohydrates, as well as some of the B vitamins that are normally associated with beef or meat products. The best natural food on the list is fresh skimmed milk at 10.5 Nutripoints. All the fat has been removed and what's left is protein, complex carbohydrates and calcium. You can use skimmed milk in cooking – add some to shepherd's pie and casseroles and other such dishes.

The major trend in milk foods, aside from the man-made foods, is that as the fat and cholesterol are reduced, the Nutripoints go up. St Ivel's Shape and Delight ranges are excellent, relatively new products, which are just as tasty as ordinary yogurt and cheese but a much better nutritional choice because of the reduced fat. For example, by the way, you can always add a dash of NutraSweet or vanilla to the virtually fat-free yogurt to give it more flavour. With fresh fruit, it makes an excellent breakfast. And, of course, it's great for cooking.

Cheese is a problem food because of its high fat content. Quark soft skimmed milk cheese gets around the fat problem and weighs in at 9.5 Nutripoints. Very low fat fromage frais is the best natural cheese choice at 8.5 Nutripoints, followed by Shape very low fat Cottage Cheese at 5.5 Nutripoints.

Near the bottom of the list you find the foods that are egg, or primarily egg, with McDonald's scrambled eggs trailing the list at − 19.5 Nutripoints, the second-lowest all-time Nutripoint score (followed only by sweetbreads at − 52 from the meat Nutrigroup).

Meat/poultry/fish: At the top of the meat Nutrigroup we find raw clams at 13.5 Nutripoints and raw oysters at 13.0 Nutripoints, but the problems with contamination of shellfish make these poor choices (thus the comment on the charts and the warning on page 139 (from the Q&A section)). The very lean red meats with their high protein and nutrient content follow the shellfish, including venison, followed by baked and grilled fishes. We're happy to see tuna in water (at 7.5 Nutripoints) rating so high, as it's such an inexpensive and readily prepared food. You'll notice that the lean beefs are right up there with the lean chicken. You don't have to eliminate red meat if you stick with the very leanest cuts, because the nutrients per calorie in beef can make it a good nutritional choice. After the lean beefs we find the lean chicken and turkey choices. As with the other Nutrigroups, as you process and add salt and fat, the Nutripoints go down. The very worst choices are fatty meats like bacon and the luncheon meats. The offal types above the recommended line all have a comment on them concerning cholesterol because, while they're high in nutrients (and thus have relatively high Nutripoint scores), they're also very high in cholesterol − and therefore are not really good nutritional choices, especially if you're concerned about cholesterol.

Personalizing the Nutripoints Programme

Thus far we've been talking about the basic Nutripoints Programme which requires 100 Nutripoints per day. This level of Nutripoints is geared to someone who requires 1,000–1,200 calories per day. This is the level of Nutripoints that we use at the In-Residence Program at the Cooper Clinic. We do so because almost all of our patients are trying to lose some weight. After they've finished two weeks at the Clinic on this level, we recommend that when they go home they move up to

Level 2 of the Program and 1,200–1,500 calories and, in some cases, 1,800 calories. In no case do we recommend that anyone go below 100 Nutripoints daily, because you really cannot expect to get adequate nutrients at this level. Moreover, such a low level of calories would have a negative effect on your metabolism.

(We don't, by the way, pinpoint the calories precisely for two reasons: first we want to de-emphasize the importance of calories as a measure of foods and, secondly, we can't specify any more precisely without losing the element of choice that you enjoy with Nutripoints.)

But this basic level of Nutripoints that we use at the Clinic isn't right for everyone. Daily nutritional needs depend on age, sex, frame size, weight and activity level: obviously a small woman who weighs seven and a half stones and who is totally sedentary is going to need fewer calories than a 200-pound football player in training.

In general, you may well find that you need fewer calories on Nutripoints than you might think. We've had many patients on the 1,000–1,200 regime who begin by thinking that they won't be satisfied with this number of calories. But, because so much of the fat is eliminated, 1,000 calories can turn out to be far more food than you might imagine. My suggestion is to begin at a level of the system that might be a bit lower than what you think your daily caloric needs are. If you find you're not getting enough food, move up to the next level of Nutripoints. There is an element of trial and error in choosing the right level for you. If, after being on one level for a couple of weeks, you find it's too much or too little food, adjust to the next level accordingly.

Here's a breakdown of the three levels of Nutripoints, so you can work out where you might need to personalize the system and adjust your daily total goals:

Level 1: 100 Nutripoints daily/1,000–1,200 calories.

This basic level of 1,000–1,200 calories per day is adequate for anyone on a weight-loss programme (which is why we use it at that level at the Cooper Clinic) or for a basically sedentary woman of 9 stones or less.

The serving recommendations are those we've already looked at:

Nutrigroup	Servings	Goal
Vegetables	4	55
Fruits	3	15
Grains	2	10
Pulses/nuts/seeds	1	5
Milk/dairy	2	10
Meat/poultry/fish	1	5
	Total:	100

Level 2: 150 Nutripoints daily/1,500–1,800 calories.

This level is appropriate for the following individuals: active women; inactive heavier women; inactive men; and men over 14 stones who are trying to lose weight.

Nutrigroup	Servings	Goal
Vegetables	6	85
Fruits	4	20
Grains	3	15
Pulses/nuts/seeds	2	10
Milk/dairy	2	10
Meat/poultry/fish	2	10
	Total:	150

Level 3: 200 Nutripoints daily/2,000+ calories.

In this level we've increased the vegetable, fruit and grain servings in order to increase the complex carbohydrates. On Level 3, you don't have to be so particular about aiming for the top of the lists to keep calories under control; there's more margin for error when you need more calories per day. But you should still avoid any foods below the recommended level.

Nutrigroup	Servings	Goal
Vegetables	8	120
Fruits	6	30
Grains	4	20
Pulses/nuts/seeds	2	10

Milk/dairy	2	10
Meat/poultry/fish	2	10
	Total:	200

Don't be overwhelmed by the number of servings for, say, vegetables, in this level of Nutripoints: you can simply increase the amounts of a serving of a single food instead of having many different foods. For example, instead of 3 oz (75 g) of sliced carrots for 1 serving and 30.0 Nutripoints, have 6 oz (150 g) for 2 servings and 60 Nutripoints. And remember that in the fruit Nutrigroup, you can have fruit juice as a serving. Many people who are on this level of Nutripoints are very active and require a significant amount of liquid throughout the day. If you ensure you drink a no-sugar-added fruit juice instead of a soft drink, this will fulfil some of your fruit servings. Instead of a Capri Sun Orange fruit drink at − 5.5 Nutripoints, have some apple juice at 2.5 Nutripoints, some orange juice at 11.5 Nutripoints, or some unsweetened grapefruit juice at 11.0 Nutripoints.

The Vegetarian Option

It wasn't so long ago that vegetarians were considered at best 'off-beat', at worst, freaks. Their image wasn't improved by fanatic converts who raged against 'murder and oppression' of animals, and thereby alienated meat-eaters and vegetarians alike. But just as people are now willing to believe that smoking can cause lung cancer and high-fat and cholesterol diets can cause heart disease, they are also willing to entertain the notion that meat may not always be the best and only source of protein in our diets. Many health organizations are saying that not only is a vegetarian diet safe (people used to worry that you couldn't get sufficient protein from it), but it can also be a healthier option than a diet that includes meat.

Solely on the basis of nutritional factors including avoidance of excessives like cholesterol and fat and in an effort to increase fibre, Nutripoints has already incorporated some vegetarian principles. We've decreased the number of recommended meat servings to one a day, and we've switched the main source of protein from meat/fish/ poultry to a combination of meat/fish/poultry plus pulses.

The advantage of getting some of your protein from plant sources rather than solely meat/poultry/fish is that, along with the protein, you're getting more complex carbohydrates, more fibre, less saturated fat and less cholesterol. As you already know, the reduction of these elements in your diet will make you less susceptible to cancer and heart disease.

In addition to avoiding the 'lifestyle' diseases, there's another factor that argues in favour of shifting the emphasis off meat as the primary source of protein in your diet: by 'eating low on the food chain', as vegetarians refer to this option, you lessen your chances of accumulating toxic substances. Any drug that livestock animals are treated with eventually ends up in their meat. A diet very high in meat is eventually introducing these toxins into your body, and no one knows what the ultimate effects of these toxins will be. In addition to toxins introduced by man in the form of drugs, animals are also more likely to harbour viruses or other diseases that can be passed to man. In general, animal diseases can be passed to us while plant diseases cannot. When you weigh up all the factors, from drug contamination to disease to contaminants such as those that regularly affect some shellfish, it seems clear that you're going from increased potential for harm to decreased potential for harm when you shift your emphasis from meat to other sources of protein.

I've been a vegetarian for sixteen years and I suppose I'm living proof of what a vegetarian diet can mean in terms of health: my cholesterol level is about 140 (3.7 mmol/l), and my best recent time on the treadmill was rated 'superior'. I also feel that my energy level is terrific, and my general state of health, excellent.

If you're interested in vegetarianism, you might want to consult some of the excellent books that have been published on the subject, including *The Cranks Recipe Book* by David Canter, Kay Canter and Daphne Swann (Grafton Books, 1985).

There are various kinds of vegetarians and here's how they are identified:

strict vegetarian or *vegan*: this is the most restricted level of vegetarianism. They eat no animal products at all, including no dairy produce and eggs.

lactovegetarians: these vegetarians eat milk, cheese and other dairy products with the exception of eggs. They also refrain from eating meat, fish or poultry.

ovolactovegetarians: these vegetarians eat animal protein in eggs and dairy products but no meat, fish or poultry. I am an ovolactovegetarian.

There is also, by the way, a new kind of vegetarian these days who doesn't eat any red meat. This isn't an official category of vegetarianism, but it's quite popular. While such people are not really vegetarians, they still represent a trend because they're avoiding a major source of fat and cholesterol, as well as any potential toxins.

The Nutripoint vegetarian option is geared to the ovolactovegetarian option, because I believe it's the safest type of diet: you're totally eliminating any flesh food – meat – but you're still getting complete protein in the form of dairy and low-fat cheese and yogurt. The protein (which many people worry about) is completely adequate at 75 g a day – clearly more than the average of 70 g recommended in the UK for men and for women per day.

Adequate protein has always been the controversial point of vegetarian diets. And many people have been put off vegetarianism because they've been worried about 'food combining'. There's something about having to worry about eating rice with beans to get certain nutrients that makes people think if they don't eat the right foods together in the precisely correct combinations, they'll wither and die. The fact is that you *do* need to pay attention to getting adequate amounts of certain foods, but this is very easy to do and it soon becomes second nature. Most importantly for many people – you don't have to combine all these foods at the *same meal*. Here's why:

The reason that animal protein is an excellent source of protein for the human body is that it contains essential amino acids that your body needs but cannot produce on its own. Foods that are high in these essential amino acids are called 'complete', or high quality. Meats are high in these amino acids because the animal has put them together from the plants it's eaten: the balance is already achieved.

Meats are therefore a 'complete' or high-quality protein. To get the balance of high-quality protein without meat, you have to do the combining yourself. Some plant foods are high in one amino acid and some are high in others: by combining them you achieve a complete protein. And, as I mentioned, you don't have to make the perfect combination at each meal; the body is far more adaptable than that. Your body has an amino acid pool that stores amino acids for future use. As long as you eat a variety of foods that complement one another within a few days of each other, you'll achieve the effect of high-quality protein.

Some examples of food combinations that provide complete protein are:

cereal with milk	rice with sesame seeds
baked beans on toast	pulse soup with bread
macaroni and cheese	corn tortillas and beans
cheese sandwich	pea soup and bread
rice/bean casserole	lentil curry with rice

Figure 1 gives a graphic summary of how to achieve complete protein with combinations of foods.

If you're starting a vegetarian diet, you should know that it will be high in fibre and you might have an adjustment period during which you'll experience excess intestinal flatulence. This is due to the fact that certain bacteria work to break down fibre and, in the process, give off gas. The body eventually adjusts and produces less gas (though it will still produce a bit more than when on a low-fibre diet), but there are various methods to cut down on this gas. When starting a vegetarian regime, I suggest you adapt your diet slowly.

First, be sure to cook all pulses thoroughly; they're supposed to be soft, and if they're too chewy they are probably undercooked and therefore likely to cause more gas. It often helps to soak pulses in plenty of water overnight, and then discard the water and add fresh for cooking. Don't eat pulses with other gaseous vegetables like cabbage. And, if you have a serious problem with gas and bloating from pulses, you might want to stick to the pulses that are least likely to cause gas – including lentils, black-eyed peas, lima beans, chick peas and white beans.

Figure 1: Summary of Complementary Protein Relationships*

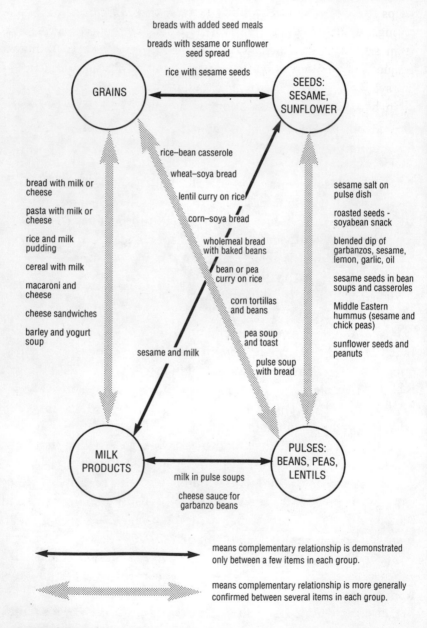

breads with added seed meals

breads with sesame or sunflower seed spread

rice with sesame seeds

GRAINS

SEEDS: SESAME, SUNFLOWER

bread with milk or cheese

pasta with milk or cheese

rice and milk pudding

cereal with milk

macaroni and cheese

cheese sandwiches

barley and yogurt soup

rice–bean casserole

wheat–soya bread

lentil curry on rice

corn–soya bread

wholemeal bread with baked beans

bean or pea curry on rice

corn tortillas and beans

pea soup and toast

pulse soup with bread

sesame salt on pulse dish

roasted seeds - soyabean snack

blended dip of garbanzos, sesame, lemon, garlic, oil

sesame seeds in bean soups and casseroles

Middle Eastern hummus (sesame and chick peas)

sunflower seeds and peanuts

sesame and milk

MILK PRODUCTS

PULSES: BEANS, PEAS, LENTILS

milk in pulse soups

cheese sauce for garbanzo beans

means complementary relationship is demonstrated only between a few items in each group.

means complementary relationship is more generally confirmed between several items in each group.

* Adapted from Frances M. Lapé, *Diet for a Small Planet*

You might also notice that your body produces more frequent and looser bowel movements while on a high-fibre diet. This is actually good: your digestive system is getting waste out of your body as quickly as possible, and the fibre is absorbing water which helps dilute carcinogens and excrete them. Ensure you have enough to drink. More frequent bowel movements also keep fat from sitting in the colon and causing a cancer risk. In addition, frequent bowel movements are helping to flush cholesterol out of the system.

So, here's the vegetarian option for the 1,000–1,200 calorie version of Nutripoints:

Nutrigroup	Servings	Goal
Vegetables	4	55
Fruits	3	15
Grains	2	10
Pulses/nuts/seeds	2	10
Milk/dairy	2	10
	Total:	100

You'll notice that this version of the vegetarian option simply substitutes one additional pulse serving for the meat/poultry/fish option. If you prefer, instead of the two pulse servings, you can have one pulse serving and one milk/dairy serving.

The 1,500–2,000 calorie version is:

Nutrigroup	Servings	Goal
Vegetables	6	85
Fruits	4	20
Grains	4	20
Pulses/nuts/seeds	3	15
Milk/dairy	2	10
	Total:	150

The 2,000+ calorie vegetarian option is:

Nutrigroup	Servings	Goal
Vegetables	8	120
Fruits	6	30
Grains	4	20
Pulses/nuts/seeds	3	15
Milk/dairy	3	15
	Total:	200

As with the other, higher-calorie versions of Nutripoints, you don't always have to depend on a huge number of servings from one Nutrigroup: you can sometimes simply increase the serving sizes to double the Nutripoints in a single serving. And you can get some of your vegetables, as well as fruits, in juices.

Nutripoint Recovery

I have always found that a great limitation of a traditional 'diet', which was most commonly a weight-reduction diet, was that you had to stick pretty strictly to the prescribed food choices and menus. This is not a whim of the diet-creators; in the best diets it's done to ensure that you get an adequate balance of protein/carbohydrates/fat and that you get sufficient nutrients. (Of course, there are many terrible diets around that ignore this important concept entirely, but that's another story!) In order for these diets to fulfil their promise of weight loss *and* adequate nutrition, they had to insist on strict compliance with the recommended menus.

Of course, what this meant in practical terms was that once you 'cheated' and put butter on your toast or ate a biscuit, you were lost. You'd failed. Most people felt that following such a diet was walking a tightrope: one slip and they might as well throw in the towel. Patients had often presented their 'diet histories' as a series of failed diets. Or else they would lose some weight on a particular diet, and then 'go off' the diet and gain it all back. Or gain it back with interest.

Nutripoints is different. It puts the control back in your hands because it puts the information in your hands. You don't have to rely on a menu plan or a list of food choices devised by someone else; you make the food choices you like. And if you follow the system, you'll achieve your goal.

And what about these 'failures'? They don't exist on Nutripoints. That's because you have the means to *quantify* your food choices yourself. This doesn't mean that you won't sometimes get fewer Nutripoints than you should, or perhaps too few or too many servings in one or more of the Nutrigroups. But when you do stray from the system, you can recover. Because Nutripoints are numbers. If you get fewer points on one day, you can re-double your efforts on the next day and get a higher score.

I tread lightly here because some people look upon the recovery feature of Nutripoints as a licence to binge. In other words, they think that if they get 200 Nutripoints on Tuesday, they can go wild on Wednesday and get only 10 Nutripoints and still be on top of things: the extra 100 Nutripoints on one day will help make up for the missing 90 the next. It doesn't work this way.

The basic premise of Nutripoints is that you want to improve your nutrition and your health. You know that it's not good to eat three slices of bacon and two fried eggs. Even if you eat the best diet in the world the following day, that overload of fat and cholesterol and sodium is going to take its toll. No system can tell you that it won't. The difference with Nutripoints is that if you don't reach your goal one day, you can still recover the next by trying harder.

The way I explain this to my patients is that they don't have the licence to eat a bowl of ice cream. But, if they find themselves at a dinner party and the main course is crab cooked in lots of mayonnaise with broccoli in cheese sauce and chocolate pie for dessert, they don't have to refuse to eat. They can eat some of their meal, working on getting a low Nutripoint score for that day, and move on the next day to choose from the tops of the Nutrigroups so that their daily 'atonement' score will be particularly high. They'll be helping their bodies by making an extra effort to reduce the fat, cholesterol and calorie intake that was exceeded the previous day.

Because Nutripoints is a numbers system, it gives you the power to improve your overall nutritional status when circumstances have forced you into a situation where your score is low.

Shopping for Nutripoints

Now that you know where you stand before you embark on the Nutripoints Programme, I hope you're inspired to jump right in. You can start immediately, with your next meal, if you wish. Or you can take a day or two to familiarize yourself with the lists and stock your kitchen cupboards with foods that are high in Nutripoints, while you discard those that could sabotage your score.

One patient told me, after he had been on Nutripoints for a month, that the biggest change in his life was the volume of food in his fridge. And it wasn't what you might think. Before Nutripoints, he said that his fridge frequently looked half empty. That's because it was filled with processed and frozen prepared foods. After all, a box of frozen carrots in butter sauce doesn't take up as much room as a bunch of fresh carrots. And a frozen pie doesn't take up as much room as some fresh chicken and fresh vegetables. He says now, after Nutripoints, when he opens his fridge he sees the colours of real foods instead of lots of packages. And his fridge always looks jammed.

Here are some tips on shopping that will help you through the supermarket maze:

Prepare to shop

1 Amazingly enough, *a high percentage of all food purchases are impulse buys*! This means that nearly half of what we buy is just something that looks good at the time. It may not have a good nutritional value, or it might not even fit our personal 'foodstyle'. So many of us go into a 'supermarket trance' the minute we hit the aisles and begin buying for a fantasy family. When we unload the grocery bags at home, we too often realize that we didn't get half of what we need, and what we did get we don't have much use for. The cure for this is a shopping list. Yes, it's basic, but it works. Buy only what's on your list, and perhaps other items that you regularly use and that are on special offer.

2 Pin your list up in your kitchen, perhaps attached with a magnet to your fridge door, so that every time you notice you need something, you jot it down. Take the time to check Nutripoints for

foods where you could make a substitution for a food that's higher in Nutripoints.

3 If you have some recipes that you're going to try, be sure to check them and add all necessary ingredients to your shopping list. It's amazing how often we never get around to preparing a certain recipe because we keep forgetting to buy that one crucial ingredient.

Time your shopping trips

1 Shop when your energy level is high and your temptation level low. You probably already know that you shouldn't shop when you're hungry. Don't shop when you're tired, either. One patient told me that her husband could always tell when she was exhausted: she came home from her usual after-work shopping trip with nothing but frozen meals. If you are going to buy nothing but frozen meals, at least make sure in advance that they're ones that are high in Nutripoints!

2 If at all possible, avoid taking small children to the supermarket with you. It's terribly distracting to have to argue with a three-year-old who wants sweets and sugared cereals and keep your mind on your list at the same time. If you must bring children with you, plan ahead and bring something – a small toy or healthy snack packed in an old margarine tub – that will keep them occupied. One patient told me that she got her two children to help out at the supermarket: she would instruct them to find certain items they were familiar with and praise them lavishly when they did. They enjoyed helping and were distracted from the usual supermarket temptations.

3 Frequent the biggest and best-stocked supermarket in your area. I recommend that you look for a supermarket with the best and most extensive produce section and adopt it as your regular shopping place. The advantage of frequenting the same supermarket is that you can develop a relationship with the manager and request that they carry certain items. Some high-Nutripoint frozen meals, for example, might not be available in your local shops but, if you request them, many managers will be happy to stock them.

Shop wisely

1 Buy fresh fruits and vegetables in season. They're almost invariably tastier and more nutritious.
2 Never buy junk foods! Never! If you have them in the house you'll probably eat them. Many people use guests as an excuse to buy things they'd never have around ordinarily. If you're having guests, prepare snacks and meals that are high in Nutripoints. They'll enjoy them as much as you do, and you'll be doing them a favour by sparing them the chip and dip route! If you must have some kind of snack food around, buy it in the smallest possible size and, if possible, individual packages.
3 If you're buying convenience foods, make sure they're high in Nutripoints.

Eating Out

Many of my patients ask me for tips on dining out. I wish I could evaluate all the various restaurant preparations, so I could give you Nutripoints for each menu entry, but because of the endless variations in restaurant recipes, even for the exact same items, that's impossible. What this means is that a familiarity with the Nutripoint charts will help guide your food choices so you can maintain your optimal diet. But, to some degree, without Nutripoints to guide you, you're back into the old days of watching fats, etc. in order to eat well. Here are a few general tips that should help you eat well in restaurants.

- If possible, choose the restaurant in advance. And choose a place that you know has some good Nutripoint choices on the menu. If you become a regular, many restaurants will be happy to fulfil certain requests, such as a vegetable combination dish that's not on the menu, or plain grilled fish or meat that they would ordinarily cook with butter. We're lucky today in that many restaurants have responded to consumer demand and become health-conscious: they offer plain grilled or baked foods, salads without dressing, vegetarian dishes and low-fat starters routinely.

- Chinese, Japanese and Indian restaurants are good choices for restaurants that tend to serve healthy foods. They use plenty of grains and vegetables, and the meat or fish portions of the meals tend to be relatively small.
- If you're with a group that's ordering cocktails, stick with a carbonated soda water with a twist of lemon. Or perhaps a Virgin Mary or another mixed drink without alcohol. An orange juice spritzer of half carbonated water and half orange juice is refreshing, and a good nutritional choice.
- If the restaurant puts bread and rolls on the table, unless others at your table object, ask them to remove the butter. It's too easy to find yourself smothering a piece of roll with butter or dabbing it on your potatoes or vegetables. You'll find that good crusty rolls and bread really don't need butter, and the savings in terms of calories and cholesterol will be well worth it. And if the restaurant doesn't serve the bread warm, you can always ask them to heat it because this brings out the natural flavours and makes it more satisfying.
- Always be sure to order salad without dressing. As we've seen, salad dressings can be a major source of fat and cholesterol if they're made with cheese or cream. Have your salad with just a bit of olive oil and vinegar, or ask if the restaurant has a low-fat or low-calorie dressing option.
- Be sure to order special dishes in advance when travelling by air. The fruit, vegetarian, or diabetic options that many airlines offer are excellent choices giving a delicious fresh meal that's largely free of excess fat and sodium.

Here are some tips for specific kinds of restaurants:

Chinese: Chinese food can be an excellent choice, as it relies on lots of vegetables cooked quickly to retain nutrients. Stir-frying is a terrific method of cooking that most Chinese restaurants rely on. It uses very little oil, and therefore adds little fat to the foods. Most Chinese vegetable and fish dishes are good choices. The only drawback of Chinese restaurants is their liberal use of monosodium glutamate (which some people are allergic to) and their use of salty and/or sugary sauces. Whole steamed fish with sauce on the side can be an excellent choice, and simple stir-fried chicken and vegetable dishes are also good. The white or brown rice that help to round out the meal are good choices, as are the following selections: mixed vegetables, won ton soup, steamed dumplings. But avoid foods like crispy fried beef, fried won tons, and any sweet and sour dishes.

French: French food can be difficult because of the use of sauces. If you stick with plain grilled meat or fish and simple salads, you'll be fine. Avoid anything prepared remoulade because that refers to a mayonnaise sauce. Be sure to steer clear of vichyssoise and other cream-based soups, and onion soup with cheese on top. (You can ask for the onion soup without the cheese as an alternative.) Clear soups are the best choices. Stick with green salads, and ask them to serve the dressing on the side. The bread is fine but, again, avoid the butter and stay away from croissants, which are loaded with butter. The best dessert bets include fresh fruits, and pass by the cream!

Indian: Indian restaurants provide some excellent choices because of their traditional reliance on pulses, vegetables and yogurt-based sauces and dips. Some of the foods that are particularly good choices on an Indian menu include dhal, vegetarian curries, raita, pulka (unleavened bread), basmati rice with vegetables, lentil soups, and tandoori baked chicken (which has been marinated in yogurt and roasted). Avoid the chapati (fried bread), samosa (fried appetizers), and any food served with muglai (creamy curry sauce) or any coconut milk curry sauce. Be sure to avoid egg-based dishes. The biggest problem with Indian food is that many restaurants use ghee (which is clarified butter) or coconut oil (one of the few vegetable products that is a saturated fat) for cooking. Be sure to ask about this; many restaurants will use other oils for cooking if you so request.

Japanese: Japanese restaurants can offer a good array of choices high in Nutripoints. The cuisine of Japan is low in fat and makes good use of a variety of vegetables. Miso soup is a good choice as it's based on soya with vegetables. Udon (noodles) served with broth and various meats and vegetables is a good main course, as are the yakitori (chicken or beef) preparations which are meats grilled on a skewer. Be sure to avoid any fried dumplings and any smoked or pickled foods. Tempura, which is fried, is not a good choice. And avoid tonkatsu (fried pork) and torikatsu (fried chicken). And, because of problems with seafood contamination, be very careful that the sushi you eat is from a highly reputable restaurant that serves only the freshest fish from the best sources.

Italian: We traditionally think of Italian food as being heavy – and it can be. But the fact is that southern Italian cuisine is now recognized as among the healthiest in the world. You just have to be careful to avoid northern-Italian-style cuisine, which is rich in fat and cream sauces. Cioppino (seafood soup) is a good appetizer, as is minestrone soup. Steamed mussels in a red sauce can make an appetizer or a meal. Pasta with vegetable and/or tomato sauces are good choices. Just be careful to avoid pasta selections that have cream-based sauces or ones that are loaded with cheese. Avoid fettucini Alfredo, lasagne (except vegetable lasagne), cannelloni and garlic bread. Plain grilled fish or meats can be good choices.

The Perfect Match: Boosting Your Nutrition

Good nutrition depends on careful shopping, careful food storage, the best cooking techniques, and also on the chemistry of the foods themselves as they work in your body. The absorption of certain nutrients can be improved when certain foods are eaten in combination; conversely, some foods inhibit the availability of nutrients when eaten with certain other foods. Alcohol, for example, impedes the body's absorption of various vitamins and minerals including thiamin, calcium, Vitamin D, folic acid and Vitamin B12. Here are some other examples, adapted from the very informative American text, *Jean Carper's Total Nutrition Guide*, on how you can get the best nutritional value from your foods by mixing and matching:

- Boost your iron absorption – and this is particularly important for women – by adding Vitamin C to any meal or food that's rich in iron. Just one glass of orange juice can boost the absorption of non-haeme (non-meat) iron by 200 to 500 per cent!
- Avoid drinking tea with meals. Excess tea can help induce iron-deficiency anaemia. It takes only two mugs of strong tea to reduce the amount of non-haeme (non-meat) iron you can absorb with a meal.
- White wine can boost the absorption of iron from a meal, while red wine contains tannins that can inhibit it. This is not to encourage consuming wine, as it can destroy nutrients and has to be detoxified by the body. But if you must have wine, white is a better choice.
- Megadoses of Vitamin C can impair Vitamin B12 absorption to the point where a deficiency can develop.
- Fruits and vegetables that are high in potassium (including spinach, bok choy, tomatoes and cantaloupe melon) can help counter the effect of excess sodium in the diet; this can be helpful for people who have a genetic disposition to hypertension.
- Many medications block or inhibit the absorption of various nutrients. Antibiotics, for example, can have an effect on your absorption of Vitamins K and B12. If you take medication regularly, including the contraceptive pill, check with your doctor to see if that medication has any effect on your nutritional status.
- Never add baking soda when cooking vegetables, as the alkaline solution thus created can destroy water-soluble vitamins like riboflavin (Vitamin B2) and Vitamin C.

Common Questions About Nutripoints

I've tried, in the text, to cover every aspect of Nutripoints that you need to know about. But sometimes information is more accessible in a question and answer format. Also, I've been interested to discover that there are certain common questions that my patients ask that wouldn't fit into any category at all! So here are the most common questions people ask about Nutripoints.

- *Why do I want to get more rather than fewer Nutripoints? Isn't this different from traditional programmes that recommend you eat the least amount of calories?*

For some people, adjusting to a positive goal (Nutripoints) rather than a negative one (calories) takes a bit of a psychological shift. But in the long run, as my patients tell me, it's far more appealing and far easier to live with.

Yes, Nutripoints is different. A Nutripoint number assigned to a food is not, like a calorie, a one-dimensional number. Rather, it's an overall quality rating of the food that considers a number of factors – both positive and negative ones. You want to get more Nutripoints because the better a Nutripoint score, the higher the quality of a given food. The numbers are based on nutrients per calorie and the least excessives (or bad elements) per calorie. The more Nutripoints you get, the more nutrition with the least excessives.

You might think of a Nutripoint as one point towards your vitamin quotient for the day, 100 of which will give you 100 per cent of the USRDA (which exceed UK recommendations), providing the points are distributed over the six Nutrigroups.

- *What happens if you eat too many points for the day or for one Nutrigroup?*

If you stick with the recommended number of servings for each Nutrigroup, you can't get too many Nutripoints. Anything over the 100 Nutripoints for the day or the goal for a given Nutrigroup is that much more nutrition you are concentrating into the food you eat. And remember that this 'excess' good nutrition is fine, because you are getting it in a natural form; it's nothing like taking megadoses of vitamins.

There is one problem with getting too many Nutripoints within one group. In some Nutrigroups, the only way to get super-high levels of Nutripoints (while staying within the recommended number of servings) is to pick most of your servings from the very top of the list.

If you do this, it's at the expense of variety which, I must stress, is very important.

Remember that each food has a 'fingerprint' of nutrients that distinguish it from other foods. If you chose all your servings in vegetables from, say, turnip tops, you won't be diversifying your portfolio of vitamins and minerals. It would be much better to get one serving of turnip tops and the other servings from vegetables below turnip tops, but still within the recommended area of the list.

- *If I eat more than 100 Nutripoints for the day, doesn't that mean that I've eaten too many calories?*

Remember, the higher the Nutripoint score, the higher the density. This means, the more nutrition per calories. A high Nutripoint score means that you are getting a higher quality of food while the number of servings you have determines the number of calories. If you get 300 Nutripoints, within the recommended number of servings, you'll be within calorie limitations and the quality of your food will be excellent.

- *How do you work out your score for a food item that's listed in the charts for more or less than you ate of that item? For example, if you eat a whole roast beef sandwich but the points are only given for half a sandwich, what do you do?*

Whether the points are negative or positive points, you double them if you eat double the portion listed. But don't forget that you must count that food item as *two* servings from that Nutrigroup. If you eat half the portion listed, you get half the Nutripoints and you count that food as a half a serving.

You'll notice that some foods list portion sizes that may be half of what you'd expect. This is a tip-off that the food is calorie-dense. A large-portion size is a sign that the food is a low-calorie, high-quality food as it takes so much volume to fulfil the calorie requirement for a serving.

- *What happens if I eat more than the recommended number of servings per day?*

There are two purposes to having a recommended number of servings per day. First, they provide the formulation within the

Nutrigroups for balance between the different vitamins and minerals. Secondly, they provide the proper mix of carbohydrates, protein and fats for the overall daily totals. After you pick the Nutripoint level that suits you (see page 99), if you eat any more than the recommended number of servings, you will not be guaranteed your level's caloric limit.

The point I make over and over to my patients is this: when you stay within the recommended boundaries of Nutripoints, everything works. When you abandon those boundaries, you have to begin to worry about all the old problematic factors – including calories, cholesterol, sugar, fat, sodium, etc.

- *If I can get my 100 Nutripoints in one serving before I fulfil the serving requirements either for a Nutrigroup or for the day, why should I eat more food and more calories?*

There are two components to an optimal diet: one is total calories and the other is the right mix of carbohydrates, fat and protein. Even though you had a good start by eating a food high in Nutripoints, you won't achieve all the requirements of your body unless you eat at least the specified number of servings per day. The goal of Nutripoints is to pick the highest-quality foods within each group that you like, thus getting all your calories or thus limiting your calories to the right amount, *while at the same time* providing the proper mix of carbohydrates, protein and fat as well as the highest level of other nutrients, including vitamins and minerals.

- *What if I just try to eat foods that are high in Nutripoints and don't bother with the serving requirements?*

To get the full benefit of Nutripoints, you must consider the serving requirements along with the food scores. Think of it this way: the food scores take care of getting the best; the serving requirements take care of limiting the worst. If you just pay attention to getting foods with high scores, your nutritional status will no doubt be improved. But that's only half the picture. You still need to limit the excessives, including fat, saturated fat, cholesterol, sugar, sodium, alcohol and caffeine. Nutripoints can only assure you of achieving all these goals if you follow the system as it was designed: high food scores in conjunction with the correct serving requirements.

- *I'm forced because of business to eat out a lot. What if I can't get in my pulse serving for a day because I can't find anything appropriate on a restaurant menu?*

This is a common problem – even if you don't eat out at restaurants. Many people are simply not used to buying and cooking pulses. Indeed, I've assumed that you won't be able to get in the pulse serving every day, and I've allowed for it by occasionally substituting a meat/poultry/fish serving in its place.

If you miss a serving from the pulse Nutrigroup, the best alternative is to substitute a serving from the meat/poultry/fish Nutrigroup. Naturally, you should try to make your substitution from the top of that Nutrigroup. You'll want to get at least a 5-Nutripoint meat/poultry/fish serving so that your total in the meat Nutrigroup for that day would be 10 rather than 5. This substitution will ensure that you're getting adequate protein for the day without too many extra calories.

- *What would happen if I occasionally ate a few foods from below the recommended line? What, really, is the reason for a cut-off point?*

If you dip below the recommended levels on the charts, it will be more difficult to achieve the goals of the system, and it will be impossible to guarantee the results promised by Nutripoints. If you try to balance a poor choice with foods that are very high in Nutripoints, it will help you regain your balance. But it's possible that the poor food choice is so high in one of the excessives that it totally causes you to exceed the limit for that excessive. Your other good choices are therefore limited in how much they can redeem you: they can give you optimal nutrients for that day, but they can't take away the excessive amounts of whatever excessive you've eaten.

- *What if I'm short in Nutripoints for one Nutrigroup but over the goal in another: is that OK?*

There's one simple answer for many questions about Nutripoints: once you abandon the programme, you forfeit what it promises. I don't mean to make this sound bleak. It's just that the system has been designed to work as it's laid out. Once you begin to modify it, results can't be guaranteed. This doesn't mean that you need to abandon hope if you are short of a few Nutripoints. The fact is that most people find that they're eating better than they've ever eaten before in their lives on Nutripoints, even if they don't follow the system religiously. So, in answer to the above question, it's impossible to say what your status would be if you were short in one Nutrigroup. If you were short by just a few points, you're probably OK. If you're short in one or two Nutripoints every few days, you're less likely to be OK.

- *If you go over your Nutripoint goal for the day – say you get 200 Nutripoints – how bad could it be to eat a food with a – 3, which only pulls your score down a little bit?*

It's difficult to appreciate at first why it's so important if you cut a few points off your daily score, unless you understand how the numbers and servings function as *limits* as well as guidelines. If you eat a negative food when you've achieved a high Nutripoint score for the day, it means that, while you've achieved all your *essential* goals, you haven't stayed within your *excessive* limits. In other words, you've probably eaten too much fat and/or cholesterol, and/or sugar, and/or sodium, and/or calories. So while you've acquired all your vitamins and minerals, you could be harming yourself by consuming, say, too much cholesterol. You can more easily understand why this would be so just from a logical standpoint. Would it make logical sense for someone to get a high Nutripoint score – say 350 Nutripoints – and then eat 150 points worth of negative foods to get their final score down to 200? Of course not!

- *Why is there so much difference between the ratings from one Nutrigroup to another? In other words, why is the highest-rated vegetable 79.0, while the highest dairy product is only 20.0 Nutripoints? Does this mean we'd be better off eating just vegetables, or does it mean that a different standard was used for different Nutrigroups?*

The same standard – the Nutripoint formula – was used to rate *all* foods. And we can see from the ratings that, in general, vegetables offer more nutrition per calorie than milk and dairy products. So you can compare foods from Nutrigroup to Nutrigroup *in general*. But you can't finally say that because vegetables are better foods, that's all you're going to eat. Balance is a crucial part of an optimal diet, and the only way to achieve balance is to choose foods from different Nutrigroups. The reason for this is that each Nutrigroup has its own nutrient profile which distinguishes it from every other Nutrigroup. And, though we know a great deal about the nutrients in foods, there are probably things yet to be discovered concerning micronutrients. Given this, there may be micronutrients in, say, grains, that your body requires to function. So, even though a grain food has a lower score than a vegetable food, you'll be avoiding grains to your peril. The only situation where foods from different Nutrigroups can be interchangeable is between pulses/nuts/seeds and meat/poultry/fish. And that's because the basic nutrient profile that seems crucial to the human body concerns protein. As it's possible to get sufficient protein from plant sources, it's possible to make exchanges from these two Nutrigroups.

- *How can all the complex information we have about vitamins and minerals be reduced to one number? How can you compare apples and oranges? Aren't oranges high in Vitamin C while bananas are high in potassium? Can't you eat carrots because they're high in Vitamin A?*

While it is true that certain foods are high in specific nutrients, many of our beliefs about eating a certain food for the sake of a certain nutrient reveal more about our past inability to compare foods accurately than about the food's usefulness.

In fact, while there are about fifty nutrients, including water, that are needed daily for optimum good health, the list can be narrowed down for practical purposes to the ten most important or 'leader' nutrients. If you are certain to consume these leader nutrients, the other forty or so will be present in sufficient amounts to meet your nutritional needs. A study was done that demonstrated this. The study tried to discover if foods rated solely on eight vitamins and minerals (protein, Vitamin A, Vitamin C, niacin, riboflavin, thiamin, iron and calcium) were valid guides to improved food choices. The foods were analysed in various ways, and finally demonstrated that nutrient density scores, even when based on only eight nutrients, do in fact serve as valid indicators of the overall nutritional worth of a food. They also found that high-nutrient density scores are a good measure of the nutritional complexity of a food. *Foods with the highest scores are high not just for one or two nutrients, but for most nutrients.* Of the fifty foods in this study, for example, forty-three had high scores for six or more of the eight nutrients measured. Foods in the middle of the ratings had good scores for only two to five of the eight nutrients measured, and most of the bottom fifty foods failed to have a decent score for even a single nutrient.

In fact, nature, with the help of Nutripoints, has made it easy for us: you don't have to eat two dozen different foods to cover all the major and minor nutrients: you just have to eat foods that are high in Nutripoints and all your nutritional bases will be covered.

- *How did you arrive at the line that defines the recommended level in the lists? Why isn't it just the point at which the numbers become negative, which seems more logical?*

The Nutripoint scores for foods had to take into account not only the absolute value of each individual food, but also how that food would fit into the pattern of balance in a daily diet. The numbers are not intended to reflect a perfect gradient; there's no point at which a food becomes taboo. My effort was as much as possible to eliminate the excessives and promote the essentials. It's all a question of relative values. So, as you reach the bottom of the lists, the food choices simply become comparatively poorer. If you choose too many of those poor foods, you won't meet the goals of Nutripoints. So the recommended line reflects an effort to guide your choices to a point where you can still choose near the bottom of the list but above the *recommended level* and still achieve your Nutripoint goals.

As to why the cut-off point is not simply all negative numbers: there are some foods that are negative but are OK to eat sometimes. Fat, for example, can be a part of your diet, but all the fats have negative numbers.

- *Why is it that sometimes there may be several foods with the same rating? Are they all exactly the same?*

When we worked out the Nutripoint scores, we carried out the numbers to the nearest one-hundredth fraction. This means that a food might have, for example, ended up with a rating of 4.26. To avoid confusion with too many numbers – and also from a practical standpoint because these differences are really quite minor – we rounded off these numbers. The food rated at 4.26 would have become 4.5.

If there are a number of foods listed as the same number, the order of listing reflects the small fractional differences in their ratings. They are listed in descending order so the first food that appears at 4.0 is better than the last food at 4.0. But remember that these differences are so minor that, for practical purposes, any food at 4.0 can be considered equal.

● *Is a food with a score of twenty twice as good as a food with a score of 10?*

Yes and no. Yes, it is twice as nutritious per calorie when adjusting for the negative factors – the excessives – that help determine the ratings. But no, it may not have double the nutrition. A food with a score of 10 may have nearly as much nutrition as a food with a score of 20, but the lower score may reflect the presence of negative factors that drop the rating. So a food with a rating of 20 is twice as good as a food with a rating of 10, *based on the criteria we have set in the Nutripoint formula.*

● *If a food has negative Nutripoints, does that mean it contains no nutrition?*

Not necessarily. A food with negative Nutripoints may contain no nutrition plus some excessives that pull it down, or it may be extremely nutritious but be pulled down by lots of excessives. You can't tell just by looking at the Nutripoint number. In these cases, its negative score is used to tell where it stands in comparison to other foods.

● *If something has 100 Nutripoints, does that mean it's a perfect food?*

Not necessarily. It's possible that a food with an extremely high Nutripoint rating is high in nutrition per calorie, but it doesn't mean that it's perfectly balanced over the eighteen essentials that we look at. There really is no perfect food. Good nutrition comes from a balance – a balance that you achieve by choosing from the six Nutrigroups.

- *Are you absolutely positive that I'll get 100 per cent of my required vitamins and minerals if I get 100 Nutripoints per day?*

If you get 100 Nutripoints per day you can be reasonably well assured that you're getting 100 per cent of your requirements for all the essential vitamins and minerals. If, however, you make many of your food choices from near the bottom of the lists, it is possible that you will occasionally be slightly below 100 per cent on some of the nutrients. The system has to take this very small risk if it's to allow you to make the food choices yourself. If you try to choose many of your foods from the higher portion of the list, you'll have no trouble getting 100 per cent of your requirements. And if you get over 100 Nutripoints, there's no doubt that you'll be reaching, and probably surpassing, your requirements for all the essential vitamins and minerals.

- *Why are some foods that are high in cholesterol at the top of the list? I thought cholesterol was a negative factor and would therefore pull that food's score down.*

You'll notice that there are some foods near the top of the list, particularly in the meat/poultry/fish Nutrigroup, that have a symbol identifying them as a high cholesterol food. What this means is that these foods, though high in Nutripoints, are also high in cholesterol. This occurs because these foods are extremely high in vitamins and minerals. They earned their scores honestly according to the Nutripoint formula. But their cholesterol level is, none the less, extremely high.

Most of the foods that fall into this category are offal such as liver. Liver acts as a storage system in the body to store vitamins and minerals, and that's why it's so rich in nutrients. But it also produces cholesterol – about 70–80 per cent of cholesterol is produced by the liver; the rest is from dietary sources. About 1,000 mg of cholesterol is produced by the human body each day. As animal livers also produce cholesterol, if you eat liver, you're eating a concentrated source of cholesterol. By the way, not all offal is rich in nutrients, and the Nutripoint charts reflect this. Sweetbreads, for example, are offal, but they're not high in nutrients – and you'll find them at the very bottom of the meat/poultry/fish list.

Another reason that liver, despite its high nutritional content, may not be a good food choice is that one of the functions of the liver is to detoxify the bloodstream. Any contaminants that are in the body are processed by the liver, and that organ therefore becomes a concentrated source of such toxins which, obviously, are not a positive element in any diet.

All foods on the Nutripoints list above the recommended line that are high in cholesterol have daggers (†) next to them. By 'high in cholesterol' I mean foods that have a cholesterol per calorie ratio of 1.0 or above; or, in other words, for every calorie there is 1 or more mg of cholesterol. From a practical standpoint, this means that, while these foods are high in nutrients, they should be avoided — despite their high Nutripoint scores. Just one 3 oz (75 g) serving of lamb's liver, for example, would have approximately 400 mg of cholesterol, which would put you well above the American Heart Association guidelines of 300 mg of cholesterol per day.

● *What about the fact that oxalic acid, which is a component of green, leafy vegetables, binds the calcium in greens so that it is not available and not readily absorbed by the body? Do you take this sort of thing into account in the formula?*

While it's true that oxalic acid does interfere to some degree with the absorption of calcium by the body, it doesn't have as negative an effect as some people believe. Certain foods do contain oxalic acid, and this acid can combine with calcium and magnesium to form insoluble compounds which are thus unavailable to the body. But most foods simply don't contain enough oxalic acid to bind with any significant amount of calcium or magnesium in the food. Thus green, leafy vegetables can still be considered a good source of calcium in the diet when supplemented with a variety of low-fat dairy products.

Different absorption levels could not be taken into account in the Nutripoints formula because there are simply so many variables connected with absorption that couldn't be quantified. In the section on food combinations (page 115), however, you'll find some helpful information on how you can boost absorption of nutrients. Also, the section on essentials (page 59) will give you tips if you're concerned about a particular nutrient.

- *How does the Nutripoint Programme assure me that I get my citrus fruit, green leafy and yellow/orange vegetables every day?*

The beauty of Nutripoints is that it automatically fulfils the requirements we've heard from nutritionists over the years. The reason we've had citrus fruit so highly recommended is that it's very high in Vitamin C. But Nutripoints also identifies other foods that are high in Vitamin C. If you choose foods from the top of the list, you'll be getting foods, citrus or not, that are probably very high in Vitamin C.

As for the green/leafy or yellow/orange vegetables, Nutripoints identifies these vegetables very highly in the first place. These foods are high in Vitamin A. (Green leafy vegetables are also high in Vitamin C and calcium.) The Vitamin A that you get from yellow/orange vegetables is in the form of beta carotene, which we've been hearing so much about recently. The body does not care whether it gets its beta carotene from green leafy vegetables or yellow/orange vegetables. Either one will fill the bill. Picking foods high on the Nutripoint lists will assure you that you're getting foods high in all your vitamin/mineral requirements.

Remember that it's an old-fashioned concept to assign one vitamin or one mineral to a single food. Nature has made it easy for us, as Nutripoints reveals: most foods that are generally high in one vitamin or mineral are also high in others. In other words, the good foods are usually very good, and the bad (or unnatural) ones are awful!

- *How does getting 100 Nutripoints assure me that I'm eating sufficient vitamins and minerals, and limiting calories, cholesterol, sodium, sugar, caffeine and alcohol?*

The formula for Nutripoints does this by identifying foods that are simultaneously highly nutritious as well as low in the excessives. Foods that appear below the recommended level are really the other half of the equation because, if you avoid them, you'll be steering clear of foods that would put you over the limit on any one of the excessive factors. Together – avoiding the negative and getting the positive – you achieve your goal.

- *How can you say that following the programme will meet or exceed recommendations of the American Dietetic Association, the American Heart Association, the American Cancer Society and the National Cancer Institute?**

* Similar recommendations are given in the UK by the DHSS.

The American Dietetic Association officially recommends the use of the USRDAs for every adult. Nutripoints is designed to fulfil these requirements. The American Dietetic Association also makes the following recommendations and you'll readily see that each of these recommendations is reflected in the Nutripoint formula:

1 eat a variety of foods;
2 maintain a desirable weight;
3 avoid fat, saturated fat and cholesterol;
4 eat foods with adequate starch and fibre;
5 avoid too much sugar;
6 avoid too much sodium
7 if you drink alcohol, do so in moderation.

The American Heart Association recommends a limit of 300 mg cholesterol per day, and a limit of 3,000 mg of sodium per day. The recommended limits are part of the formulation of Nutripoints and are the limits set in the formula.

The American Heart Association also recommends 30 per cent less fat consumed as calories in the diet as a preventive measure against many types of cancer, particularly colon and breast cancer. Nutripoints sets 30 per cent of fat as calories as the upper limit in its formulation.

The American Cancer Society recommends getting a high level of Vitamins A and C from foods, since these vitamins have been correlated with lower rates of cancer. This is one of the strengths of Nutripoints: it identifies foods highly concentrated with Vitamins A and C, and thus is a cancer-prevention diet.

The National Cancer Institute recommends 25–35 g of dietary fibre per day. Nutripoints sets 35 g as the recommended amount per day in its formulation.

Picking foods from the top of the Nutripoint lists could result in a diet that betters these various guidelines.

● *Will the Nutripoints Programme help prevent cancer?*

There are still many questions about the causes of cancer. But there's no doubt that there are steps you can take in terms of nutrition that will decrease your risks for certain types of cancer. Nutripoints will certainly lower your risk for various types of cancers, as it incorporates the basic recommendations of the American Cancer

Society into the tenets of the system. These seven recommendations include:

1 avoid obesity;
2 cut down on total fat intake;
3 eat more high-fibre foods;
4 include foods rich in Vitamins A and C in your daily diet;
5 include cruciferous vegetables in your diet;
6 eat moderately of salt-cured, smoked or nitrite-cured foods;
7 keep alcohol consumption moderate, if you do drink.

You'll recognize that each of these recommendations is reflected in the basic Nutripoints formula.

• *Does your system take into account the nutrient losses from transportation, storage and cooking?*

In general, no. It's simply impossible to account for all these factors with the exception of cooking. You'll notice that many of the fresh foods are listed raw and also cooked. This will give you an idea of how the nutrition might vary from one state to another, though sometimes the variation is simply a reflection of amounts. Raw cabbage, for example, has greater volume than cooked cabbage.

But the effects of transportation and storage are too variable and can't be measured. Some of these issues are discussed on page 45.

• *Why did you put certain things like lemons in the condiments section when they would seem more logically to be in the fruit section?*

Most of the items in the condiments group are the foods that you'd expect to find there, including spices and seasonings. Other foods are listed there because they're normally eaten in such small quantities that the calorie level for a given portion would be less than 20. This means that they couldn't logically fit into the regular fruit Nutrigroup because the serving size would have to be so large that it simply wouldn't make sense. The average number of calories for the portions in the fruit Nutrigroup are 50–100. For lemons to fit there, I'd have to suggest that you eat two whole lemons to count as a serving. So a quarter of a lemon at 5 or 6 calories fits logically in the condiment section. Also, in the condiment section I've adjusted the calorie portion of the formula so that the portion sizes fit normal eating patterns.

- *Why do you include foods like pulses in your system? Many people never eat them! And why is Nutripoints geared towards massive amounts of fruits and vegetables?*

As a bank robber replied when asked why he robbed banks: 'Because that's where the money is.' Pulses, fruits and vegetables are highly nutritious foods, and they should play a large role in our daily diet. It's unfortunate that pulses are unfamiliar to many people (though I think that's changing). Pulses are an excellent source of protein, with no cholesterol, lots of fibre and plenty of complex carbohydrates. If we replaced one quarter to one half of our meat consumption with pulses (and the Nutripoints Programme is designed to do this), we would be avoiding the major causes of the most prevalent 'lifestyle' diseases – including cancer and heart disease.

As to the massive amounts of fruits and vegetables, again, that's where the nutrients are! One of the major revelations of Nutripoints is that the best value in nutrition lies in fruit and vegetables. That's where we get the most nutrition for the fewest calories. The bonus of fruit and vegetables in terms of nutrition is that these foods are also high in complex carbohydrates and simple *bulk*: if you're dieting, they fill you up while giving you good nutrition. This is the exact opposite of junk foods: they *don't* fill you up and give you *nothing* in terms of good nutrition.

- *What about combination foods like lasagne that have meat and a grain and a vegetable in them – how did you determine which Nutrigroup to put them in?*

You'll notice that I've categorized combination foods according to the major component either by volume or calories, whichever made more sense. In the case of lasagne, it's in the grain Nutrigroup, because the largest ingredient is the pasta. I couldn't break down these combination foods because manufacturers only provide data for the whole dish, and not the parts of the dish.

- *Does the Nutripoint formula take into account food additives and contaminants?*

No, it doesn't. I would love to be able to do so, but there simply is no reliable, standardized way of measuring these elements in various foods. (For a fuller discussion of this subject, see page 43.)

- *How did you gather your data?*

About half of my information was from the Cooper Clinic Data Base, which is based on USDA information. A vast quantity of money went into the research behind these formulations. I feel it's the most reliable data available. In their analyses they give the number of samples they tested, and the range is usually from 10 to 200. That means for some bits of information – say the amount of Vitamin A in a carrot – they might have tested 200 carrots. In most cases, they've done enough to assure its accuracy. But in an occasional case I found some margin for error. For example, in a few instances, I found data that was based on only one sample by the USDA. This single sample disagreed with data from either a manufacturer or from another source. In those cases, I followed common sense and used my own judgement to ascertain which data made the most sense. For each food, I've examined between one and four sources to corroborate evidence.

With brand-name foods and fast foods, I've had to rely on manufacturers. In most instances, manufacturers send samples to reliable and creditable laboratories to get their nutritional data. In most cases, these manufacturers sent me copies of the reports as they came from the laboratories, or else they gave the name of the laboratory or research company. Some manufacturers don't have their foods analysed, and have no nutritional data whatsoever. Some manufacturers based nutritional information for their products on the USDA data for basic foods, and extrapolated to arrive at their own 'analyses'. Whenever there was doubt or inaccuracy or contradiction, I sifted through the available evidence to come up with what I believe is the most fair and accurate interpretation of the data.

- *Foods are constantly changing. How can you keep up with brand names and fast foods that come out after your list was compiled?*

It's true that food formulations change constantly. But I am continually adding to the original foods, and I'd like to solicit manufacturers to send me information on their new foods – especially if they're formulating 'light' or healthier foods. We'd love to include such foods in new editions of Nutripoints. (I'd also like to think that, with the advent of Nutripoints, manufacturers will have all the more reason to create healthier foods. If consumers know which foods are better for them, surely it's an incentive to buy. And there's nothing like consumer pressure, or the pressure of the market place, to convince manufacturers to create ever-healthier formulations of foods.)

- *Why are supplemental foods rated higher than natural foods? For example, I noticed that most of the cereals that are fortified have much higher scores than the natural, unfortified cereals. I thought you believed in getting vitamins naturally.*

Yes, I do believe in getting vitamins naturally. That's why we have an asterisk next to a food that is significantly fortified. 'Significantly fortified' means that 50 per cent or more of the nutrition comes from fortification. In these cases, when foods are highly fortified, we have to take a look at the basic food that existed before the fortification. For example, Kellogg's All Bran is basically a good food. Everything from the whole wheat is there, including the fibre and other basic nutrients. The fortification is added on top of something real. But if you look at Kellogg's Rice Crispies, you'll see a different story. In that case, there's little basic food at all. You simply have to use common sense. If Rice Crispies is the only thing your children will eat, you could do worse. (Though I do believe it's best to avoid such foods right from the begining, so children don't get used to them.) And, by the way, a helpful way to judge a cereal that's highly fortified, and therefore high in Nutripoints, is to check the ingredients listed on the box: if sugar is listed near the beginning of the ingredients list, you'll know that the cereal is highly sweetened and, despite the fortification, not a good nutritional choice.

- *What about oysters and clams? I notice they're high on the list, but are they good food choices?*

While it's true that oysters and clams are high on the list, you'll notice that they're marked with a double dagger (‡) indicating caution. I had to grant them their high number of Nutripoints because that's how the system worked out. They're very high in certain minerals, including calcium, iron, zinc, phosphorus and potassium. But, in fact, I don't believe that they're particularly good food choices because of the problems with shellfish contamination.

- *What if someone doesn't have problems with cholesterol, high blood pressure, or weight control but wants to achieve good nutrition? Your system has a built-in bias against cholesterol, sodium, sugar and fat – but surely foods that are high in these things can also be very nutritious?*

Nutripoints rates the food, not the eater! Foods that are highly rated are the best available for the body based on today's scientific research. We know that excess cholesterol, excess sodium, excess sugar and fat are not good for the body. If you're lucky enough not to have a problem with any of the lifestyle diseases today, that unfortunately does not mean that you won't be facing them tomorrow. A prudent diet is also a *preventive* diet. Everybody has an 'excessive threshold' that seems to allow them to consume a certain amount of foods that aren't good for them. But then they reach a point where they're trying to reverse a problem like high blood pressure, or excess weight or diabetes. A prudent diet, one that follows Nutripoints, is going to protect you in the future as well as make you feel well today.

- *Is Nutripoints for everyone?*

Nutripoints is primarily for healthy adults. It's not designed for anyone under the age of eighteen who might need additional calcium and protein in their diet. Nutripoints is designed for people who are sedentary to moderately active, with no special medical problems that might involve diet. It's wise to check with your doctor if you have any medical condition that might require special attention before you embark on the Nutripoints Programme.

- *Can I follow Nutripoints if I have food allergies?*

If you have any particular medical condition, you should consult your doctor before beginning Nutripoints. A doctor or nutritionist could help you adapt Nutripoints to suit your particular condition.

- *Is there a Nutripoint Programme for children or people with special needs, like pregnant women or athletes?*

No, not at present, although we're working on just such a programme. We hope in the future to come up with various versions of Nutripoints that will accommodate people with special needs.

- *How is Nutripoints used at the Aerobics Center in the In-Residence Program?*

At the Aerobics Center, Nutripoints is used primarily as a weight-loss programme and a total-nutrition programme for those who want to maintain their weight. In the future, we'll have a version of Nutripoints specifically geared to weight loss for the general public; this book is geared to every healthy adult who wants to improve their level of nutrition, though many people find that they lose weight using Nutripoints as it's outlined in this book, particularly if their diet was generally poor.

- *Why didn't someone think of Nutripoints before?*

It took the happy marriage of computer technology with the latest nutritional data to produce Nutripoints. I have to assume that it wasn't done before because it never occurred to anyone that it *could* be done. Point systems had been designed that rate foods. But no one had developed a system that so exhaustively quantifies every element of a food, plus puts it into a total system that assures optimum nutrition. And certainly no nutrition plan has ever been offered that allows you complete freedom to choose, given only the limitations of the foods' Nutripoints scores.

- *Do you use the Nutripoints Programme yourself?*

Yes I do. I kept a diet diary for two weeks before I began using Nutripoints. As a nutritionist and a vegetarian, my diet was already good: low in fat, high in fibre, and high in vitamins and minerals. But my diet survey revealed that I was getting between 150 and 200 Nutripoints daily and about 1,500 to 2,000 calories. Now, with Nutripoints, I'm getting between 200 and 300 Nutripoints daily, and I'm eating roughly the same number of calories.

PART 5

Nutripoint Lists

The lists that follow are in four parts:

The Nutrigroup Ratings lists show the rating of every food within its Nutrigroup, highest to lowest. There are six basic Nutrigroups:

1. Vegetables
2. Fruits
3. Grains
4. Pulses/nuts/seeds
5. Milk/dairy
6. Meat/fish/poultry

There are four types of foods on the Nutrigroup Ratings lists:

1. Basic foods
2. Generic foods
3. Brand-name foods
4. Fast foods

There are also five Other Group lists:

1. Fats/oils
2. Sugar
3. Alcohol
4. Condiments
5. Miscellaneous

The following are notes and explanations concerning various aspects of the lists.

BASIC FOODS

These are just what you would think: apples, whole wheat flour, milk, chicken breast, and so on. They're foods that are unprocessed.

GENERIC FOODS

You'll notice that some of the foods on the list are neither brand names nor basic foods such as grapes. These foods are what we call *generic foods*. They have ratings based on data published by the Ministry of Agriculture, Fisheries & Food, and provided by food manufacturers and consultants. Some of these are foods that have had some processing, such as canned peas or tomato sauce; others are what are known as *home recipes*, such as coleslaw. Home recipes are standard recipes that most people would use at home to prepare certain foods.

BRAND-NAME FOODS

These are foods that have been processed by a particular manufacturer who also provided the nutritional information used as the basis of analysis of these foods. These foods include everything from Bird's Eye frozen spinach to Wrigley's chewing gum.

FAST FOODS

These are foods that are served by fast-food restaurants, and we've tried to include the most popular items on their menus, from salads, to burgers, to pizzas.

You'll notice that there are three columns for the food ratings. The *Nutripoints* column, obviously, is the rating of the food.

The *Food Name* column, of course, identifies the food.

The *Serving Size* column shows the amount of food that is rated. The measurements include pieces, millilitres, grams, tablespoons, and teaspoons. Various explanations concerning serving sizes appear in the text.

Next to a food name you'll sometimes find an asterisk (*), a dagger (†), or a double dagger (‡). An asterisk means that the food is fortified, a dagger indicates that it contains too much cholesterol, and a double dagger warns the reader to exercise caution when eating a food because it may contain contaminants.

FORTIFICATION

You'll notice, particularly in the grain Nutrigroup, that many of the foods have an asterisk (*). This means that these foods derive at least 50 per cent of their nutritional value from fortification. There are further discussions of this topic in the text (see page 132), but I'll simply reiterate here that some controversy exists about the value of fortification. Often, nutrients have been removed through processing and then replaced artificially. While these foods do contain large amounts of certain nutrients, they're not 'natural' in that they aren't as nature formulated them. In general, the fortified foods at the top of the list are far preferable to fortified foods lower on the list because the top foods (cereals usually) begin with a whole food and then fortify it. The foods lower down sometimes have sugar as a primary ingredient, with vitamins and minerals added to that. My basic suggestion concerning fortified foods is that if you choose them, check the labels to be sure that the food is based on a real, basic food. One of the best tip-offs to a fortified food with little value is if the label contains any of the various terms for sugar (see page 79) listed among its first few ingredients.

CHOLESTEROL

Some foods, particularly those in the meat/poultry/fish Nutrigroup, have a dagger (†) indicating cholesterol. Again, this has been discussed more fully in the text (see pages 73, 125), but briefly, the notation means that these foods have a content of cholesterol per calorie of 1 milligram or more. This is a high concentration of cholesterol and, whatever the ranking of the food, I suggest that you avoid foods with the cholesterol mark.

CAUTION

Some shellfish have a double dagger (‡), which indicates the possibility of contamination. While many of these foods are high in Nutripoints, care must be taken when eating them.

NUTRIPOINT FOOD RATINGS
Vegetable Group

Nutripoints	Serving Size		Food Name
79.0	150	g	TURNIP TOPS, Boiled
75.0	100	g	SPINACH, Raw, Chopped
72.5	150	g	BOK CHOY, Raw, Shredded
57.0	175	g	SPINACH, Whole Leaf, Fz, Bird's Eye
54.5	50	g	PARSLEY, Fresh
53.5	175	g	SPINACH, Fresh, Cooked
53.0	100	g	BROCCOLI, Raw
52.5	20	pc	WATERCRESS
46.0	100	g	BROCCOLI SPEARS, Frozen, Bird's Eye
44.0	8	pc	ASPARAGUS, Fresh
42.5	2	pc	PEPPERS, Sweet, Red, Raw
42.5	150	g	SPINACH, Frozen, Cooked
42.0	175	g	SWISS CHARD, Cooked
41.5	125	g	BROCCOLI, Caul & Red Peppers, Fz, Bird's Eye
40.5	125	g	TOMATOES, Canned, Peeled, Drained, Prince's
40.5	100	g	CAULIFLOWER, Raw
40.0	75	g	BRUSSELS SPROUTS, Cooked
39.0	100	g	CABBAGE, Common, Raw, Shredded
38.5	175	g	BROCCOLI, Cooked
38.5	125	g	KALE, Chopped, Cooked
37.5	2	pc	GREEN PEPPER, Raw
37.5	125	g	CAULIFLOWER, Cooked
35.5	175	g	CHICORY GREENS, Raw
35.5	1	pc	CARROTS, Raw
34.0	100	g	LETTUCE, Butterhead/Boston/Bibb, Chopped
33.0	125	g	SALAD, Tossed, No Dressing
32.5	75	g	MUSHROOMS, Fresh
32.5	8	pc	ASPARAGUS, Canned
31.5	175	g	CABBAGE, Common, Chopped, Cooked

Nutripoints	Serving Size		Food Name
31.0	100	g	OKRA, Cooked
30.0	1	pc	TOMATO, Fresh
30.0	75	g	CARROTS, Sliced, Cooked
29.5	75	g	CABBAGE, Red, Raw, Shredded
29.0	100	g	RADISHES, Raw
28.0	75	g	PEAS AND CARROTS, Frozen, Cooked
27.0	75	g	BRUSSELS SPROUTS, Frozen, Cooked
27.0	8	pc	ASPARAGUS, Frozen, Boiled
26.0	100	g	OKRA, Raw
25.0	75	g	PEAS AND CARROTS, Canned
24.5	75	g	CABBAGE, Savoy, Raw, Shredded
24.5	150	ml	JUICE, V-8 Vegetable
24.5	150	g	KOHLRABI, Raw
24.5	150	ml	JUICE, Tomato
24.5	125	g	RUNNER BEANS, Boiled
24.0	10	pc	SPRING ONIONS
23.0	175	g	CAULIFLOWER, Frozen, Bird's Eye
23.0	125	g	TOMATOES, Canned
22.0	75	g	VEGETABLES, Mixed, Canned
21.5	125	g	SALAD, Tossed, with Tomato
20.0	8	pc	CELERY, Raw
20.0	75	g	CUCUMBER, Raw
20.0	4	T	TOMATO PURÉE, Canned
19.5	150	g	TURNIPS, Cooked
19.0	100	g	MUSHROOMS, Cooked
18.5	125	g	LETTUCE AND TOMATO
18.0	50	g	KELP
18.0	75	g	TURNIPS, Raw
18.0	10	pc	LETTUCE, Iceberg
18.0	100	g	VEGETABLES, Mixed, Frozen, Cooked
18.0	100	g	VEGETABLES, Mixed, Frozen, Bird's Eye
17.5	75	g	ALFALFA SPROUTS, Raw

Nutripoints	Serving Size		Food Name
17.5	125	g	SAUCE, Tomato, Canned
17.0	75	g	BAMBOO SHOOTS, Raw
17.0	250	g	SAUERKRAUT, Canned
17.0	100	g	AUBERGINE, Cooked
17.0	125	g	BROCCOLI, Corn & Red Pprs, Fz, Bird's Eye
16.5	125	g	BAMBOO SHOOTS, Canned
16.0	2	pc	LEEKS, Raw
16.0	175	g	COURGETTES, Raw
15.5	100	g	BEANS, Green, Cut, Frozen, Bird's Eye
15.0	175	g	COURGETTES, Cooked
15.0	150	ml	JUICE, Carrot
14.0	125	g	ASPARAGUS, Cuts, Canned, Green Giant
13.0	225	g	SOUP, Vegetable, no Salt
13.0	275	g	MUSHROOMS, Canned
13.0	100	g	BROCCOLI, Caul & Crts, Cheese Sauce
13.0	200	g	BEANS, Green, Whole, Canned
12.5	1	pc	ARTICHOKE, Cooked
12.0	0.5	pc	SWEET POTATO/YAM, Baked
12.0	250	g	SOUP, Vegetable
11.5	100	g	PARSNIPS, Raw
9.0	100	g	POTATOES, Canned
8.5	75	g	ONION, Raw
8.5	50	g	SHALLOTS, Raw
8.5	0.5	pc	POTATO, Baked
8.5	75	g	PARSNIPS, Cooked
8.0	75	g	CORN, Frozen, Cooked
8.0	75	g	CELERIAC, Raw
7.5	100	g	LEEKS, Cooked
6.0	100	g	CORN, Sweet, Frozen, Bird's Eye
6.0	0.5	pc	CORN ON COB, Fresh, Cooked
5.5	25	g	POTATO POWDER, Instant, Tesco's
5.5	50	g	FLOUR, Potato

Nutripoints	Serving Size		Food Name
5.5	100	g	WATER CHESTNUTS, Canned
5.0	125	g	CORN W/RED AND GREEN PEPPERS, Canned
4.5	125	g	CORN, Creamed, Canned
4.5	250	g	SOUP, Vegetable Beef
4.0	75	g	SALAD, Spinach, w/Eggs/Bacon/Tomato
4.0	150	g	SAUCE, Spaghetti, Meatless
3.5	225	g	SOUP, Minestrone
3.0	60	g	ARTICHOKE HEARTS, Marinated
3.0	50	g	COLESLAW
2.5	125	g	CORN, Whole Kernel, Canned, Green Giant
2.5	250	g	SOUP, Tomato
2.5	100	g	VEGETABLES, Japan. Style, Fz, Bird's Eye
2.5	50	g	POTATOES, Au Gratin
2.0	225	g	SOUP, Vegetable, Campbell's
2.0	50	g	POTATOES, Scalloped
2.0	50	g	CAULIFLOWER CHEESE, Marks & Spencer's
2.0	50	g	POTATO, Instant Powder, Made Up
1.5	250	g	GAZPACHO
1.0	125	g	SOUP, Cream of Asparagus
1.0	50	g	POTATOES, Mashed, Home Recipe
1.0	4	pc	FRENCH FRIES
0.5	225	g	SOUP, Tomato, Campbell's
0.5	125	g	SOUP, Potato
0.5	1	T	PICKLE, Sweet, Heinz
0.0	5	pc	CRISPS, Potato
−0.5	2	pc	ONION RINGS, Fried
−0.5	125	g	SOUP, Cream of Celery
−0.5	0.25	pc	McDONALD'S REGULAR FRENCH FRIES
−0.5	50	g	CAULIFLOWER, Fried w/Breadcrumbs
−1.0	75	g	POTATO SALAD, Home Recipe
−1.0	25	g	MUSHROOMS, Fried w/Breadcrumbs
−1.0	75	g	SOUP, Cream of Mushroom

Nutripoints	Serving Size		Food Name
−1.0	100	g	SOUP, Cream of Tomato, Canned, Heinz
−1.0	50	g	SOUP, Cream of Mushroom, Campbell's, Low Sodium
−1.5	250	g	SOUP, Onion
−1.5	2	T	KETCHUP, Heinz
−2.0	0.5	pc	McDONALD'S HASHBROWN POTATOES
−2.5	75	g	RHUBARB, Cooked, with Sugar
−2.5	0.25	pc	PIE, Rhubarb, Homemade
−2.5	225	g	SOUP MIX, Cream of Mushroom, Cup-A-Soup
−2.5	225	g	SOUP MIX, Tomato, Cup-A-Soup
−2.5	100	g	KENTUCKY FRIED CHICKEN MASHED POTATOES
−3.0	75	g	SOUFFLÉ, Spinach
−3.5	225	g	SOUP, French Onion
−4.5	100	g	SOUP, Cream of Mushroom, Campbell's

Fruit Group

Nutripoints	Serving Size	Food Name
29.0	0.25 pc	MELON, Cantaloupe
21.0	1 pc	GUAVA
20.5	0.5 pc	PAPAYA
19.0	150 g	STRAWBERRIES, Fresh
19.0	75 g	CURRANTS, Black
17.5	0.5 pc	MANGO
17.0	1 pc	KIWI FRUIT
17.0	150 g	STRAWBERRIES, Frozen, Unsweetened
16.0	6 pc	LITCHI, Fresh
15.5	125 g	MANDARIN ORANGES, Canned, Unsweetened
14.0	0.25 pc	MELON, Honeydew
14.0	125 g	PLUMS, Canned, Unsweetened
13.5	1 pc	ORANGE, Fresh
13.5	3 pc	APRICOT, Fresh
13.0	1 pc	TANGERINE
13.0	0.5 pc	GRAPEFRUIT, Fresh
13.0	75 g	BLACKBERRIES, Fresh
13.0	100 g	FRUIT SALAD, Fresh
12.5	1 pc	CARAMBOLA (Starfruit)
12.5	75 g	RASPBERRIES, Fresh
11.5	6 pc	APRICOTS, Dried, Whitworth's
11.5	150 ml	JUICE, Orange, Fresh Squeezed
11.5	125 g	CHERRIES, Cooking, Stewed, no Sugar
11.0	1 pc	PEACH, Fresh
11.0	6 pc	APRICOTS, Dried
11.0	150 ml	JUICE, Grapefruit, Unsweetened
11.0	125 g	APRICOTS, Canned, Unsweetened
11.0	150 ml	JUICE, Orange, Frozen, Reconstituted
10.5	150 g	WATERMELON

Nutripoints	Serving Size		Food Name
10.5	100	g	PEACHES, Canned, Unsweetened
10.0	6	pc	KUMQUAT
10.0	225	g	FRUIT COCKTAIL, Canned, Unsweetened
10.0	1	pc	NECTARINE, Fresh
8.0	75	g	PINEAPPLE, Fresh
7.5	125	g	CHERRIES, Sour, Canned, Unsweetened
7.5	75	g	BLACKBERRIES, Frozen, Unsweetened
7.5	0.5	pc	BANANA
7.5	1	pc	PERSIMMON
7.0	150	ml	JUICE, Grapefruit, Sweetened, Canned
7.0	75	g	BLUEBERRIES, Fresh
6.5	100	g	PRUNES, Cooked, Unsweetened
6.5	1	pc	PEACHES, Canned in Juice
6.0	2	pc	PLUM, Fresh
6.0	1	pc	QUINCE
6.0	0.5	pc	PLANTAIN, Fresh
6.0	4	pc	PRUNES, Dried
5.5	75	g	PLANTAIN, Cooked
5.5	150	ml	JUICE, Grape, Unsweetened
5.5	10	pc	CHERRIES, Sweet, Fresh
5.0	2	pc	FIGS, Dried
4.5	100	ml	APRICOT NECTAR, Canned
4.5	50	g	PRUNES, Canned, Heavy Syrup
4.5	1	pc	PEAR, Fresh
4.5	50	g	GUACAMOLE
4.5	20	pc	GRAPES, Raw
4.5	1	pc	APPLE, Fresh
4.0	0.25	pc	AVOCADO, Florida
4.0	1	pc	FIGS, Fresh
4.0	40	g	RAISINS
4.0	50	g	PRUNES, Cooked, with Sugar
4.0	5	pc	DATES

Nutripoints	Serving Size		Food Name
3.5	1	pc	POMEGRANATE
3.5	125	g	PEARS, Canned, no Sugar
3.0	2	pc	PEARS, Dried
3.0	2	T	RAISINS, Thompson Seedless
2.5	125	g	APRICOTS, Canned, Heavy Syrup
2.5	150	ml	JUICE, Apple
2.5	0.25	pc	AVOCADO, California
1.0	125	g	PINEAPPLE, Canned, Heavy Syrup
1.0	125	g	FRUIT COCKTAIL, Canned, Heavy Syrup
1.0	125	g	CHERRIES, Sour, Canned, Heavy Syrup
0.0	125	g	CHERRIES, Sweet, Canned, Heavy Syrup
0.0	125	g	PEACHES, Canned, Heavy Syrup
0.0	150	g	PLUMS, Canned, Heavy Syrup
−0.5	125	g	APPLE, Stewed, with Sugar
−1.0	25	g	RAISINS, Carob-Covered
−1.0	0.5	pc	PIE, Raspberry
−1.0	0.25	pc	PIE, Mince
−1.0	150	g	PEARS, Canned, Heavy Syrup
−1.5	0.5	pc	PIE, Blackberry
−1.5	0.5	pc	PIE, Strawberry
−1.5	25	g	RAISINS, Chocolate-Covered
−1.5	0.25	pc	BANANA SPLIT
−2.0	0.25	pc	PIE, Apple
−2.0	0.5	pc	PIE, Peach
−2.0	0.5	pc	PIE, Blueberry
−2.0	0.25	pc	PIE, Fruit, with Pastry Top and Bottom
−2.0	1	T	COCONUT
−2.0	8	pc	OLIVES, Black
−2.0	125	g	SALAD, Waldorf
−3.0	100	g	PIE FILLING, Apple
−3.5	0.25	pc	CHERRY CHEESECAKE
−3.5	1	pc	COCONUT, Bounty Bar

Nutripoints	Serving Size		Food Name
−3.5	25	g	COCONUT, Raw
−4.0	8	pc	OLIVES, Green
−4.0	0.25	pc	PIE, Lemon Meringue
−4.5	1	T	ORANGE MARMALADE, Chiver's
−4.5	8	pc	OLIVES, Green, in Brine
−5.0	1	T	JAM, Robertson's, All Flavours
−5.0	0.5	pc	PIE, Cherry
−5.0	125	g	GELATINE, Cherry Flavour
−5.0	1	T	JAM, Strawberry
−5.5	50	g	JELLY CUBES, Rowntree's
−5.5	150	ml	FRUIT DRINK, Orange, Capri Sun
−5.5	2	T	JELLY, Cranberry

Grain Group

Nutripoints	Serving Size		Food Name
27.0	25	g	*CEREAL, All Bran, Kellogg's
26.5	25	g	BRAN, Wheat
23.5	25	g	*CEREAL, 100% Bran w/Oat Bran, Nabisco
21.0	25	g	*CEREAL, Bran Flakes, Kellogg's
18.0	25	g	*CEREAL, Corn Flakes, Kellogg's
17.0	25	g	*CEREAL, Oat Munchies, Quaker
16.5	50	g	*CEREAL, Sultana Bran, Kellogg's
14.5	40	g	*CEREAL, Grapenuts
14.5	30	g	*CEREAL, Bran Flakes
14.0	25	g	*CEREAL, Special K, Kellogg's
14.0	50	g	*CEREAL, Bran Buds, Kellogg's
14.0	25	g	*CEREAL, Raisin Splitz, Kellogg's
11.5	25	g	*CEREAL, Rice Krispies, Kellogg's
11.5	25	g	*CEREAL, Team Flakes, RHM
10.5	25	g	WHEAT GERM
10.5	25	g	*CEREAL, Clusters, Quaker
9.0	8	pc	CRACKER, Snackbread, High Fibre Ryvita
8.5	30	g	*CEREAL, Nutrigrain-Rye & Oats w/Haz., Klg's
8.0	40	g	BEMAX
7.5	3	pc	CRACKER, Crispbread, High Fibre
6.5	40	g	CEREAL, Weetabix
6.0	1	pc	MUFFIN, Whole Wheat
6.0	30	g	*CEREAL, Ready Brek, Lyons', Not Made Up
6.0	40	g	FLOUR, Wholemeal
6.0	30	g	CEREAL, Weetaflake, Weetabix
6.0	2	pc	BREAD, Wholemeal
5.5	25	g	CEREAL, Puffed Wheat, Quaker
5.5	30	g	*CEREAL, Crunchy Nut Corn, Kellogg's
5.0	1	pc	CEREAL, Shredded Wheat, Nabisco

* Fortified

Nutripoints	Serving Size		Food Name
5.0	40	g	CEREAL, Shredded Wheat, RHM
5.0	6	pc	CRACKERS, Rye Crispbread
5.0	25	g	CEREAL, Shredded Wheat Spn Sz, Nabisco
4.5	30	g	FLOUR, Soya, Full Fat
4.5	25	g	CEREAL, Puffed Wheat
4.5	1	pc	ROLL, Wholemeal
4.5	1	pc	MUFFIN, English, with Raisins
4.5	2	pc	BREAD, Cracked Wheat
4.5	2	pc	BREAD, Pumpernickel
4.0	100	g	RICE, Brown, Cooked without Salt
4.0	2	pc	BREAD, Whole Rye
4.0	1	pc	MUFFIN, English
4.0	2	pc	BREAD, Wheat Germ
4.0	3	pc	BREAD, Mix Grain, Mighty White
4.0	1	pc	BREAD, Pitta, Whole Wheat
4.0	40	g	CEREAL, Creusli, Alpen
4.0	1	pc	WAFFLES
4.0	125	g	RICE, Spanish
3.5	2	pc	BREAD, Wheat, Stone Ground
3.5	25	g	MACARONI, Dry
3.5	75	g	MACARONI, Cooked, no Salt
3.5	25	g	*CEREAL, Alpen
3.5	125	g	LINGUINE, Spinach High-Protein, Buitoni
3.5	3	pc	BREAD, Hi-Fibre, Vitbe
3.5	1	pc	ROLL, Rye
3.5	6	pc	BREADSTICKS
3.5	35	g	CEREAL, Oatmeal, Raw
3.5	35	g	CORN MEAL, Dry
3.5	1	pc	BREAD, Pitta
3.5	75	g	NOODLES, Spinach, Cooked
3.0	75	g	SPAGHETTI, Cooked

* Fortified

Nutripoints	Serving Size		Food Name
3.0	4	pc	CRACKER, Crispbread Dark Rye, Ryvita
3.0	60	g	LINGUINE, Buitoni
3.0	0.5	pc	PIZZA HUT PEPPERONI PAN PIZZA
3.0	1	pc	ROLL, Cracked Wheat
3.0	100	g	RICE, White, with Added Salt
3.0	0.5	pc	BUN, Hoagie
3.0	6	pc	CRACKERS, Wheat Crispbread, Starch Red.
3.0	8	pc	CRACKER, Whole Wheat
3.0	40	g	CEREAL, Frosties, Kellogg's
3.0	100	g	RICE, White, Cooked, w/o Salt
3.0	1	pc	MUFFIN, Bran
3.0	40	g	FLOUR, Plain White, Household
3.0	30	g	FLOUR, White
3.0	2	pc	BREAD, French
3.0	2	pc	BREAD, Rye, Light
3.0	40	g	BULGAR, Dry
2.5	2	pc	BREAD, Italian
2.5	125	g	LASAGNE, Cooked
2.5	0.5	pc	ROLL, French, Part Cooked
2.5	4	pc	BREAD, Nimble
2.5	2	pc	BREAD, White
2.5	1	pc	BREAD ROLL, White, Crusty
2.5	1	pc	BREAD, Soda
2.0	3	pc	BREAD, White, Toasted
2.0	100	g	RICE, Pilaf
2.0	25	g	NOODLES, Egg, Whole Wheat, Uncooked
2.0	25	g	CEREAL, Puffed Rice
2.0	1	pc	BUN, White Hamburger
2.0	1	pc	BAGEL
2.0	100	g	CEREAL, Porridge Oats, Quaker Scotts
2.0	40	g	BREADCRUMBS
2.0	1	pc	ROLL, White

Nutripoints	Serving Size		Food Name
2.0	1	pc	ROLL, Starch Reduced

Nutripoints	Serving Size		Food Name
1.5	1	pc	BUN, Hot Dog
1.5	150	g	RAVIOLI, Canned in Tomato Sauce
1.5	40	g	CEREAL, Coco Pops, Kellogg's
1.5	4	pc	CRACKER, Rice Cake
1.5	60	g	EGG NOODLES, Cooked
1.0	0.5	pc	PIZZA, Large 16" Veggie
1.0	6	pc	BREADSTICKS, Garlic
1.0	0.5	pc	PIZZA, Large 16" Ham
1.0	0.5	pc	LASAGNE, Italian Cheese, Fz, Wt Wtchr's
1.0	75	g	FETTUCINI, Cooked
1.0	1	pc	PIZZA, Cheese, Deluxe, Frozen
1.0	1	pc	PANCAKE, Buckwheat
1.0	5	pc	NACHOS, Cheese/Hot Peppers
0.5	125	g	PASTA SALAD
0.5	1	pc	PANCAKE, Whole Wheat
0.5	1	pc	PANCAKE, Plain
0.5	1	pc	PANCAKE, with Fruit
0.5	1	pc	GRANOLA BAR, Chewy Choc Chip
0.5	10	pc	CRACKER, Rice, Small
0.5	60	g	PIZZA, Cheese & Tomato, Homemade
0.5	15	pc	TORTILLA CHIPS
0.5	30	g	WATER BISCUITS
0.5	1	pc	PIZZA, Thick Crust, Frozen
0.5	100	g	PUDDING, Milk
0.0	50	g	MACARONI CHEESE
0.0	25	g	POPCORN, Cooked with Oil
0.0	1	pc	BREAD, Garlic
0.0	1	pc	GINGERBREAD
−0.5	1	pc	BREAD, Banana
−0.5	200	g	SPAGHETTI, Canned in Tomato Sauce

Nutripoints	Serving Size		Food Name
−0.5	25	g	CORN CHIPS
−1.0	8	pc	CRACKER, Ritz
−1.0	0.5	pc	PIZZA, with Sausage
−1.5	100	g	STUFFING
−1.5	4	pc	COOKIES, Lemon Creme
−1.5	30	g	CRACKERS, Cream
−1.5	1	pc	TURNOVER, Fruit
−1.5	2	pc	COOKIES, French Vanilla Creme
−2.0	30	g	BISCUIT, Chocolate, Full Coated
−2.0	1	pc	GRANOLA BAR, Oats 'n Honey
−2.0	30	g	CEREAL BAR, Choc Chip Chewy, Jordon's
−2.0	30	g	BISCUITS, Plain Digestive
−2.0	0.5	pc	CAKE, Coffee
−2.0	30	g	FRUITCAKE, Plain
−2.0	0.5	pc	CHOCOLATE ECLAIR
−2.0	2	pc	COOKIES, Macaroon
−2.5	0.5	pc	DANISH PASTRY
−2.5	1	pc	CROISSANT
−2.5	40	g	CAKE, Madeira
−2.5	30	g	SHORTBREAD
−2.5	30	g	COOKIES, Sandwich Biscuit
−2.5	1	pc	FRENCH TOAST
−3.0	40	g	DOUGHNUT
−3.0	1	pc	PIE CRUST
−3.0	0.5	pc	DOUGHNUT, Jam
−3.0	0.5	pc	DOUGHNUT, Custard Filled
−3.0	30	g	COOKIES, Filled Wafer
−3.0	0.5	pc	CAKE, German Chocolate
−3.0	0.5	pc	CAKE, Devil's Food
−3.5	0.5	pc	CAKE, Dutch Apple
−3.5	1	pc	BREAD, White Fried
−3.5	30	g	CAKE, Sponge, Jam Filled

Nutripoints	Serving Size		Food Name
−3.5	0.5	pc	CAKE, Sponge, with Icing
−3.5	1	pc	COOKIES, Chocolate Chip Oatmeal
−3.5	1	pc	CUPCAKE, without Icing
−3.5	30	g	SPONGE CAKE, Chocolate, with Icing
−4.0	100	g	BREAD & BUTTER PUDDING
−4.0	2	pc	COOKIES, Chocolate Chip
−4.0	1	pc	CUPCAKE, with Icing
−4.5	30	g	ECLAIR, Chocolate
−5.0	30	g	CAKE, Sponge, Fatless

Pulse/Nut/Seed Group

Nutripoints	Serving Size		Food Name
18.0	200	g	BEAN SPROUTS, Mung, Fresh
14.0	150	g	PEAS, Frozen, Cooked
12.0	200	g	PEAS, Green, Frozen, Bird's Eye
10.5	200	g	BEANS, Mung, Green
9.0	175	g	PEAS, Black-Eyed, Canned
8.5	125	g	BEANS, Kidney, Red
8.5	150	g	BEANS, French, Boiled
8.5	175	g	PEAS, Black-Eyed, Cooked
8.0	150	g	LENTILS, Split, Boiled
8.0	175	g	PEAS, Processed, Canned, Tesco's
8.0	100	g	PEAS, Split, Boiled
8.0	75	g	BEANS, Garbanzo, Cooked
7.5	125	g	BEANS, Baked, in Tomato Sauce
7.5	25	g	SOYBEANS, Dry
7.5	175	g	PEAS, Canned
7.0	125	g	SOYBEANS, Cooked
6.5	125	g	BEANS, Pinto, Cooked
6.5	220	g	BEANS, Baked, in Tomato Sauce, Top Crop
6.5	125	g	PEAS, Sweet, Canned, Green Giant
5.5	150	g	BEANS, Baked, in Tomato Sauce, Heinz
5.5	215	g	SOUP, Lentil
5.0	125	g	TOFU
5.0	250	g	SOUP, Bean, Black
5.0	100	g	BEANS, Chilli
4.5	250	g	SOUP, Lentil, with Ham
4.5	40	g	SEEDS, Sunflower, Unsalted
4.0	250	g	SOUP, Pea
4.0	200	g	SOUP, Minestrone, Homemade
3.5	2	T	DIP, Bean

Nutripoints	Serving Size		Food Name
3.5	250	g	SOUP, Bean
3.5	125	g	BEANS, Boston Baked
3.0	125	g	CHILLI WITH LENTILS, Vegetarian
3.0	125	g	BEANS, with Pork
2.5	225	g	SOUP, Green Pea, Campbell's
2.0	25	g	TRAIL MIX
2.0	0.5	pc	SANDWICH, Peanut Butter, Whole Wheat
1.5	125	g	SALAD, Three Bean
1.5	25	pc	PEANUTS, Oil Roasted, Unsalted
1.5	0.5	pc	SANDWICH, Peanut Butter, White
1.5	25	g	SESAME BUTTER (TAHINI)
1.5	1	pc	VEGEBURGERS, Frozen
1.5	12	pc	CASHEWS, Dry Roasted, Unsalted
1.5	18	pc	ALMOND KERNELS
1.5	25	g	CASHEWS, Dry Roasted, Unsalt., Planter's
1.5	25	g	PEANUTS, Dry Roasted, Unsalt., Planter's
1.0	25	pc	PEANUTS, Oil Roasted, Salted
1.0	25	g	PEANUTS, Dry Roasted, Salted, Planter's
1.0	1	T	PEANUT BUTTER, Unsalted
1.0	25	g	MIXED NUTS, Dry Roast, Unsalted
1.0	25	g	PINE NUTS
1.0	1	T	PEANUT BUTTER, Low Sodium
1.0	25	g	BUTTERNUTS
1.0	125	g	CHILLI, Bean/Beef
1.0	25	g	MIXED NUTS, Oil Roasted, Salted
1.0	25	g	PISTACHIOS, Raw
1.0	25	g	PEANUTS, Cocktail, Planter's
0.5	1	T	PEANUT BUTTER
0.5	25	g	CASHEWS, Dry Roasted, Salted
0.5	225	g	MILK, Non-Dairy, Soy
0.5	1	T	ALMOND BUTTER, Salted

Nutripoints	Serving Size	Food Name
0.5	25 g	CASHEWS, Oil Roasted, Unsalted
0.5	0.5 pc	SANDWICH, Peanut Butter/Jelly, Whole Wheat
0.5	0.5 pc	SANDWICH, Peanut Butter/Jelly, White
0.5	8 pc	MACADAMIA NUT KERNELS
0.5	12 pc	WALNUTS
0.5	25 g	HAZELNUTS, Oil Roasted, Salted
0.5	25 g	CASHEWS, Oil Roasted, Salted
0.5	25 g	CASHEW BUTTER, Salted
0.5	12 pc	ALMONDS, Oil Roasted, Salted
0.0	6 pc	BRAZIL NUT KERNELS
0.0	15 pc	PECAN KERNELS
0.0	40 g	SEEDS, Sesame
0.0	15 g	PISTACHIOS, Dry Roasted, Salted
0.0	1 T	PEANUT BUTTER, Crunchy
−0.5	25 g	PECANS, Oil Roasted, Salted
−1.0	25 g	PEANUTS, Yogurt-Covered
−1.0	25 g	PEANUTS, Chocolate Covered
−1.0	6 pc	ALMONDS, Chocolate-Covered
−1.5	25 g	NUTS, Mixed, w/Peanuts, Planter's
−1.5	6 pc	ALMONDS, Sugar-Coated
−3.5	0.5 pc	PIE, Pecan

Milk/Dairy Group

Nutripoints	Serving Size		Food Name
20.0	225	ml	MILK, Skimmed, Calcium Fortified, Vital
16.5	25	g	MILK POWDER, Skimmed, Drd, Fort. w/Vitamins
15.0	150	ml	BUILD UP, Made w/Skimmed Milk
14.0	225	ml	MILK, Skimmed, Calcium Fortified, Calcia
10.5	225	ml	MILK, Skimmed, Fresh Pasteurized
10.5	250	g	YOGURT, Very Low Fat, Strawberry, Shape
10.5	225	ml	MILK, Skimmed, Fortified, Vitapint
10.0	250	g	YOGURT, Very Low Fat, Strawberry, Sains.
10.0	40	g	MILK, Skimmed, Dried, Marvel
10.0	225	g	YOGURT, Very Low Fat, Black Cherry, Shape
9.5	150	g	CHEESE, Skimmed Milk Soft, Quark
9.0	150	ml	MILK, Evaporated Skimmed, Carnation
8.5	175	g	YOGURT, Low Fat, Plain
8.5	175	g	FROMAGE FRAIS, Very Low Fat
8.5	100	ml	BUILD UP, Made w/Whole Milk
8.5	200	g	YOGURT, Very Low Fat, Plain, Shape
8.0	150	g	YOGURT, Low Fat, Plain, Sainsbury's
8.0	175	g	YOGURT, Low Fat, Natural, St Ivel
7.5	225	ml	BUTTERMILK, Cultured, Eden Vale
7.0	100	ml	COMPLAN, Sweet, Made with Water
7.0	225	ml	MILK, Semi-Skimmed, Fresh Pasteurized
7.0	150	g	YOGURT, Low Fat, Plain, Eden Vale
6.5	100	ml	YOGURT DRINK, Strawberry, Yop
6.0	6	pc	EGG WHITE
6.0	225	ml	MILK, Semi-Skimmed, Fortified
5.5	150	g	CHEESE, Cottage, Very Low Fat, Shape
5.0	225	ml	BUTTERMILK, Fresh
5.0	100	ml	COMPLAN, Savoury, Made with Water
4.5	125	g	YOGURT, B'Active Set, w/Vits C, A & D, Chambourcy

Nutripoints	Serving Size		Food Name
4.0	125	g	CHEESE, Cottage, Half Fat, Sainsbury's
4.0	150	ml	CUSTARD, Made with Skimmed Milk
3.5	150	ml	MILK SHAKE, Made with Skimmed Milk, Nesquik
3.5	100	g	TOPPING, Sugar Free Angel Delight, Bird's
3.5	150	ml	DRINKING CHOCOLATE, Made with Skimmed Milk
3.0	450	ml	COCOA MIX, Hot, Sugar Free, Carnation
3.0	150	g	YOGURT, Natural, Thick Set, Sainsbury's
2.5	150	g	YOGURT, Low Fat, Hazelnut, Tesco's
2.5	113	g	CHEESE, Cottage, Eden Vale Natural
2.5	225	ml	COCOA MIX, Sugar Free, Quik, Nestlé
2.5	150	g	YOGURT, Low Fat, Raspberry, Ski
2.5	150	g	YOGURT, Low Fat, Orange, Ski
2.5	150	ml	MILK, Chocolate, Low Fat (2%)
2.0	125	g	YOGURT, Low Fat Set, w/Natural Fruit, Sainsbury's
2.0	40	g	CHEESE, Cheddar-Type, Red. Fat, Tendale
2.0	150	g	YOGURT, Low Fat, Blackcurrant, Tesco's
1.5	150	g	YOGURT, Low Fat, Fruits of the Forest, Tesco's
1.5	150	g	YOGURT, Low Fat, Blackberry & Apple, Tesco's
1.5	125	g	YOGURT, Frozen
1.5	100	g	MACARONI CHEESE, Canned
1.5	150	g	YOGURT, Low Fat, Apricot, Tesco's
1.5	225	ml	MILK, Whole, Fresh Pasteurized
1.5	225	ml	MILK, Goat's
1.5	100	g	CHEESE, Cottage
1.5	125	g	CHEESE, Cottage, Low Fat, w/Pineapple
1.0	125	g	MILK, Canned, Evaporated, Unsweetened
1.0	125	g	MILK, Evaporated, Carnation
1.0	75	g	ICE CREAM, Vanilla, Loseley's
1.0	50	g	MILK, Whole, Condensed Sweet, Nestlé

Nutripoints	Serving Size		Food Name
1.0	1	T	MALTED MILK POWDER
1.0	210	g	PUDDING, Creamed Rice, Ambrosia
1.0	100	g	FROMAGE FRAIS, Plain
1.0	225	ml	MILK, Whole, UHT
0.5	225	ml	MILK, Fresh Channel Island
0.5	50	g	CHEESE, Ricotta, Low Fat
0.5	2	T	DRESSING, Yogurt
0.5	25	g	CHEESE, Mozzarella, Low Fat
0.5	25	g	CHEESE, Grated, Parmesan
0.5	0.5	pc	CANNELLONI, Cheese, Lean Cuisine
0.5	25	g	CHEESE, Swiss, Reduced Fat, Kraft
0.0	125	g	YOGURT, Greek, Sheep's, Total
0.0	125	g	YOGURT, Thick 'n' Creamy, Sainsbury's
0.0	100	ml	CUSTARD, Bird's, Made with Whole Milk
0.0	225	ml	CHOCOLATE, Hot
0.0	125	g	YOGURT, Greek, Cow's
0.0	0.5	pc	SANDWICH, Grilled Cheese, White
0.0	100	g	CREME CARAMEL
0.0	100	g	ANGEL DELIGHT, Sugar Free, Wild Straw.
0.0	100	g	MOUSSE, Fruit Flavoured
−0.5	100	ml	MILK SHAKE, w/Whole Milk, Nesquik
−0.5	100	ml	DRINKING CHOCOLATE, Made w/Whole Milk
−0.5	100	ml	MILK, Instant Natural Malted, Carnation
−0.5	125	g	YOGURT, Low Fat, Peach
−0.5	125	g	MILK, Chocolate
−0.5	80	g	PUDDING, Tapioca
−1.0	25	g	CHEESE, Provolone
−1.0	60	g	FROMAGE FRAIS, with Fruit, Sainsbury's
−1.0	25	g	CHEESE, Edam
−1.0	25	g	CHEESE, Camembert
−1.0	60	g	ICE CREAM, Non Dairy, Neapolitan

Nutripoints	Serving Size		Food Name
−1.0	25	g	CHEESE, Gruyère
−1.0	60	g	ICE CREAM, Non Dairy, Vanilla, Soft Scoop
−1.5	100	g	OMELETTE, Spanish
−1.5	0.5	pc	EGG McMUFFIN, McDonald's
−1.5	25	g	CHEESE, Mozzarella
−1.5	25	g	CHEESE SPREAD, Plain
−1.5	0.25	pc	EGG McMUFFIN, with Sausage, McDonald's
−1.5	25	g	CHEESE, Gouda
−1.5	2	T	CREAM, Non-Dairy, Imitation, Lq (Veg Oil)
−2.0	25	g	CHEESE, Romano
−2.0	50	g	CHEESE, Ricotta
−2.0	25	g	CHEESE, Cheddar
−2.0	25	g	CHEESE, Danish Blue
−2.0	0.5	pc	CAKE, Cheese, with Fruit Topping
−2.0	125	g	EGGNOG
−2.0	25	g	CHEESE, Brie
−2.0	25	g	CHEESE, English Cheddar
−2.0	25	g	CHEESE, Cheshire
−2.0	25	g	CHEESE, Double Gloucester
−2.0	75	g	MILK, Sweetened Condensed, Carnation
−2.5	25	g	CHEESE, Feta
−2.5	50	g	QUICHE, Cheese & Egg w/Wholemeal Pastry
−2.5	25	g	CHEESE, Caerphilly
−2.5	50	g	ICE CREAM, Dairy, Vanilla
−2.5	0.5	pc	BURGER KING VANILLA SHAKE
−2.5	50	g	QUICHE LORRAINE
−2.5	50	g	QUICHE, Cheese and Egg
−2.5	65	g	TOPPING, Dream, Bird's Made w/Skimmed Milk
−3.0	25	g	CHEESE, Dairylea
−3.0	75	g	SOUFFLÉ, Cheese
−3.0	25	g	CHEESE SPREAD, Pasteurized Processed
−3.0	0.5	pc	McDONALD'S CHOCOLATE MILK SHAKE

Nutripoints	Serving Size		Food Name
−3.0	50	g	CHEESECAKE, Frozen with Fruit Topping
−3.0	0.5	pc	McDONALD'S VANILLA MILK SHAKE
−3.0	25	g	CHEESE, Blue Stilton
−3.0	0.5	pc	McDONALD'S STRAWBERRY MILK SHAKE
−3.0	25	g	CHEESE, Limburger
−3.0	25	g	CHEESE, Roquefort
−3.0	25	g	CHEESE, White Stilton
−3.0	0.5	pc	SANDWICH, Egg Salad, Whole Wheat Bread
−3.5	150	ml	ICE CREAM SODA
−3.5	100	g	EGGS, Scotch
−3.5	0.5	pc	SANDWICH, Egg Salad, White Bread
−3.5	50	g	ICE CREAM, Coffee
−3.5	50	g	TOPPING, Dream, Bird's Made w/Whole Milk
−3.5	2	T	CREAM, Non-Dairy, Coffee Mate, Carnation
−3.5	0.5	pc	PIE, Custard
−3.5	50	g	CREAM, Sour
−4.0	60	g	ICE CREAM, Chocolate
−4.0	25	g	CHEESE, Neufchatel
−4.5	4	T	CHEESE FONDUE
−4.5	0.25	pc	QUICHE, Cheese/Bacon
−5.0	125	g	ICE CREAM, Butter Pecan
−5.0	2	T	CHEESE, Cream
−5.5	2	T	CHEESES, Full Fat Soft, Philadelphia
−5.5	4	T	SAUCE, Cheese
−5.5	4	T	TOPPING, Whipped
−6.0	0.5	pc	QUICHE, Cheese
−6.5	4	T	CREAM, Whipped
−7.0	2	T	CREAM, Double
−8.0	0.5	pc	EGG, Omelette, w/Ham/Cheese (1 pc = 3 Eggs)
−9.0	75	g	EGG SALAD
−10.5	1	pc	EGGS, Devilled (1 pc = Whole Egg)
−11.5	2	pc	EGG, Poached

Nutripoints	Serving Size		Food Name
−11.5	2	pc	EGG, Hard Boiled
−11.5	2	pc	EGG, Soft Boiled
−12.5	1	pc	EGG, Fried
−13.5	1	pc	EGG, Scrambled
−15.0	2	pc	EGG YOLK
−19.5	1	pc	McDONALD'S SCRAMBLED EGGS

Meat/Fish/Poultry Group

Nutripoints	Serving Size		Food Name
13.5	175	g	‡CLAMS, Mixed Species, Raw
13.0	12	pc	‡OYSTERS, Eastern, Raw
9.0	75	g	CALF'S LIVER, Fried
8.5	100	g	VENISON, Baked
8.0	150	g	CLAMS, Canned
8.0	4	pc	‡OYSTERS, Pacific, Raw
7.5	150	g	TUNA, Canned in Water
7.5	175	g	PIKE, Baked
7.5	75	g	SALMON, Steamed/Poached
7.5	100	g	HALIBUT, Baked
7.0	75	g	†LAMB'S LIVER, Fried
7.0	175	g	RED SNAPPER, Baked
7.0	150	g	TURKEY BREAST, Cured, Tesco's
7.0	175	g	BASS, Freshwater, Baked
7.0	75	g	†BEEF LIVER, Fried
7.0	175	g	COD FILLETS, Skinless, Sainsbury's Prime
7.0	75	g	OYSTERS, Grilled with Butter
6.5	125	g	TURKEY BREAST, Premium Sliced, Tesco's
6.5	75	g	ABALONE
6.5	100	g	SALMON, Canned in Water
6.5	75	g	SWORDFISH, Baked
6.5	75	g	TUNA, Fresh, Grilled
6.0	175	g	CLAMS, Steamed/Boiled
6.0	100	g	QUAIL, without Skin
6.0	175	g	HADDOCK FILLETS, Frozen, Tesco's
6.0	175	g	SOLE, Baked
5.5	100	g	PHEASANT, without Skin
5.5	100	g	STURGEON, Steamed

† Cholesterol: excessively high
‡ Caution: high risk of contamination

Nutripoints	Serving Size		Food Name
5.5	175	g	SOUP, Chicken Gumbo
5.5	125	g	PLAICE FILLET, Baked
5.5	75	g	SALMON, Baked/Grilled
5.0	75	g	CLAMS, Smoked, Canned in Oil
5.0	150	g	HADDOCK, Baked Fillet
5.0	75	g	TROUT, Baked
4.5	75	g	CLAMS, Breaded, Fried
4.5	50	g	†LIVERWURST
4.5	175	g	†CRAB, Hardshell, Steamed
4.5	3	pc	SARDINES, Canned in Oil
4.5	150	g	COD, Baked Fillet
4.5	75	g	ABALONE, Floured, Fried
4.5	125	g	HAM, Canned, Cooked, Ye Olde Oak
4.5	100	g	SMELT, Rainbow, Baked
4.5	100	g	OCEAN PERCH, Baked
4.5	150	g	WHITE FISH, in Parsley Sauce, Tesco's
4.5	75	g	TURKEY, Light Meat Baked w/o Skin
4.0	75	g	CHICKEN BREAST, Baked w/o Skin
4.0	75	g	BEEF ROUND STEAK, Lean, Grilled
4.0	0.5	pc	SANDWICH, Chicken Salad, Whole Wheat
4.0	250	g	SOUP, Beef
4.0	100	g	SHARK, Mixed Species, Raw
4.0	75	g	†BEEF HEART, Braised
4.0	100	g	SNAILS
4.0	75	g	BEEF FLANK STEAK, Lean, Grilled
4.0	175	g	TURKEY BREAST IN JELLY, Sainsbury's
4.0	175	g	SCALLOPS, Baked/Grilled
4.0	100	g	PERCH FILLET, Grilled/Baked
4.0	75	g	MACKEREL, Baked
4.0	100	g	BEEF TOPSIDE, Roast Lean
4.0	75	g	BEEF TOP LOIN, Lean, Grilled

† Cholesterol: excessively high

Nutripoints	Serving Size		Food Name
3.5	6	pc	SARDINES, Canned, Tomato Sauce
3.5	75	g	†VEAL CUTLET/STEAK, Lean, Braised
3.5	450	g	SOUP, Seafood Gumbo
3.5	75	g	FISH, Smoked
3.5	75	g	LAMB ROAST, Leg, Baked
3.5	75	g	PLAICE, BAKED
3.5	75	g	HALIBUT FILLET, Batter-Fried
3.5	250	g	BEEF STEW
3.5	0.5	pc	SANDWICH, Chicken Salad, White Bread
3.5	0.5	pc	SANDWICH, Tuna Salad, Whole Wheat
3.5	100	g	COD, Baked
3.5	75	g	BEEF TENDERLOIN FILLET, Lean, Grilled
3.5	75	g	BEEF CHUCK ROAST, Lean, Braised
3.5	75	g	TURKEY, Lt/Dk Meat, w/o Skin, Baked
3.5	200	g	TUNA NOODLE CASSEROLE
3.0	250	g	OYSTER STEW
3.0	75	g	RABBIT, Wild
3.0	75	g	TURKEY, Dark Meat, Baked w/o Skin
3.0	75	g	HAMBURGER PATTY, Lean, Grilled
3.0	175	g	BEEF, Macaroni and Tomato Sauce
3.0	0.5	pc	SANDWICH, Tuna Salad, White
3.0	75	g	LAMB SHOULDER, Lean, Baked
3.0	150	g	COD FILLET, Smoked, Poached
3.0	100	g	TUNA SALAD
3.0	100	g	PLAICE FILLETS, Baked, Gateway
3.0	150	g	SOLE FILLETS, Lemon, Fz, Sainsbury's
3.0	75	g	PORK CHOP, Loin, Lean, Baked
3.0	75	g	TURKEY ROLL, Light Meat
3.0	75	g	RABBIT, Domestic, Breaded, Fried
3.0	150	g	GROUPER, Baked
3.0	75	g	SALMON, Smoked

† Cholesterol: excessively high

Nutripoints	Serving Size		Food Name
3.0	100	g	HERRING, Grilled (Off Bone)
2.5	75	g	CHICKEN BREAST, Fried w/o Bread, w/Skin
2.5	75	g	BEEF RIB EYE, Lean, Grilled
2.5	125	g	CHICKEN FRICASSÉE
2.5	100	g	BEEF SIRLOIN, Roast Lean
2.5	1	pc	GREEN PEPPER, Stuffed with Meat
2.5	75	g	BEEF PORTERHOUSE STEAK, Lean, Grilled
2.5	175	g	LOBSTER, Steamed/Boiled
2.5	175	g	SUSHI/RAW FISH
2.5	75	g	CARP, Smoked
2.5	0.5	pc	SANDWICH, Turkey, Whole Wheat Bread
2.5	100	g	HADDOCK, Baked
2.5	75	g	CHICKEN LEG, Baked w/o Skin
2.5	75	g	BEEF T-BONE STEAK, Lean, Choice, Grilled
2.5	100	g	TURKEY, Light Meat and Skin, Baked
2.0	75	g	RABBIT, Stewed
2.0	100	g	CHICKEN SALAD
2.0	175	g	MUSSELS, Cooked
2.0	0.5	pc	SANDWICH, Chicken, Whole Wheat Bread

- -

2.0	75	g	SALMON, Baked with Butter
2.0	75	g	BEEF ROUND STEAK, Med. Fat, Grilled
2.0	75	g	CHICKEN THIGH, Fried w/o Breadcrumbs
2.0	75	g	CHICKEN Liver, Stewed
2.0	100	g	WHITING, Grilled, Baked
2.0	150	g	CHICKEN WITH DUMPLINGS
2.0	100	g	LUNCHEON MEAT, Turkey Ham
2.0	0.5	pc	SANDWICH, Chicken, White Bread
2.0	175	g	COD, Smoked
2.0	175	g	SQUID, Raw
2.0	75	g	BEEF RIBS, Baked
2.0	175	g	HADDOCK, Smoked

Nutripoints	Serving Size		Food Name
2.0	100	g	TUNA, Canned in Oil
2.0	75	g	BEEF BRISKET, Lean, Braised
2.0	150	g	BOLOGNESE, Spaghetti, Chilled, Tesco's
2.0	3	pc	CHICKEN WING, Baked w/out Skin
2.0	75	g	VEAL ROAST, Lean, Braised
2.0	0.5	pc	SANDWICH, BLT, Whole Wheat Bread
2.0	75	g	OCTOPUS, Fried
1.5	25	g	SALMON AND SHRIMP PASTE, Tesco's
1.5	25	g	SARDINE AND TOMATO PASTE, Tesco's
1.5	0.5	pc	SANDWICH, Corned Beef, Rye Bread
1.5	75	g	CHICKEN LEG, Fried, w/Skin
1.5	100	g	HERRING, Canned
1.5	75	g	DUCK, Baked, without Skin
1.5	75	g	BEEF FLANK STEAK, Med. Fat, Choice, Grld
1.5	0.5	pc	SANDWICH, Turkey, White Bread
1.5	75	g	BARRACUDA, Baked/Grilled
1.5	3	pc	BACON, Danish
1.5	75	g	CHICKEN BREAST, Fried w/o Skin
1.5	75	g	CAPON, Baked with Skin
1.5	250	g	SOUP, Chicken
1.5	75	g	HAMBURGER PATTY, Lean, Fried
1.5	75	g	EEL, Smoked
1.5	125	g	CHICKEN, Creamed
1.5	75	g	EEL
1.5	3	pc	OYSTERS, Fried
1.0	25	g	BEEF PASTE, Tesco's
1.0	25	g	CHICKEN AND HAM PASTE, Tesco's
1.0	0.5	pc	SANDWICH, BLT, White Bread
1.0	250	g	SOUP, Beef Noodle
1.0	100	g	HAM, Canned
1.0	100	g	TURKEY, Dark Meat and Skin, Baked
1.0	75	g	SCALLOPS, Fried

Nutripoints	Serving Size		Food Name
1.0	175	g	CRAB, Canned
1.0	75	g	CHICKEN BREAST, Fried w/Batter, w/Skin
1.0	4	pc	SALAMI, Pork
1.0	75	g	BARRACUDA, Breaded/Floured, Fried
1.0	125	g	HAM SALAD
1.0	75	g	PERCH, Fried w/Breadcrumbs
1.0	75	g	CHICKEN THIGH, Baked w/o Skin
1.0	0.5	pc	SANDWICH, Roast Beef, Hot
1.0	100	g	COD FISH FINGERS, Bird's Eye
1.0	75	g	BEEF SHORT RIBS, Lean, Braised
1.0	175	g	SOUP, Chowder, Fish
1.0	75	g	VEAL CUTLET, Med. Fat, Braised
1.0	75	g	SWORDFISH FILLET, Breaded, Fried
1.0	75	g	BEEF TENDERLOIN, Med. Fat, Grilled
1.0	250	g	SOUP, Beef, Heinz
1.0	250	g	SOUP, Beef & Veg, Main Course, Campbell's
0.5	2	pc	HERRING, Pickled
0.5	100	g	POUSSIN, Roast Meat Only
0.5	75	g	CARP, Baked/Grilled
0.5	50	g	PATÉ, Chicken Liver, Canned
0.5	100	g	TURKEY & HAM PIE, Tiffany's Uppercrust
0.5	75	g	VEAL ROAST, Med. Fat, Braised
0.5	0.5	pc	TURKEY POT PIE
0.5	125	g	CHOP SUEY, Beef/Pork
0.5	100	g	CHICKEN GOUJONS, Tesco's
0.5	75	g	FISH, Fried
0.5	0.5	pc	SANDWICH, Ham/Cheese, Whole Wheat
0.5	75	g	LAMB ROAST, Leg, Med. Fat, Baked
0.5	0.5	pc	BEEF POT PIE
0.5	50	g	BEEF CHUCK ROAST, Med. Fat, Baked
0.5	100	g	SALMON, Scotch Smoked
0.5	100	g	CHICKEN, Cornfed, Roast Meat Only

Nutripoints	Serving Size		Food Name
0.5	0.5	pc	CHICKEN POT PIE
0.5	4	pc	FISH FINGERS
0.5	75	g	BEEF TOP LOIN, Med. Fat, Grilled
0.5	0.5	pc	SANDWICH, Ham/Cheese, Rye
0.5	50	g	BEEF RUMP ROAST, Baked
0.5	75	g	GOAT
0.5	250	g	SOUP, Chicken Noodle
0.5	15	pc	PRAWNS, Cooked
0.0	50	g	CHICKEN FRIED STEAK
0.0	75	g	HAMBURGER PATTY, Grilled
0.0	0.5	pc	SANDWICH, Ham/Cheese, White
0.0	1	pc	CHICKEN THIGH, Meat & Skin, Baked
0.0	50	g	PORK ROAST, Baked
0.0	125	g	BEEF STROGANOFF
0.0	100	g	PORK, Sweet and Sour
0.0	0.5	pc	CHICKEN KIEV
0.0	2	pc	CHICKEN WING, Fried w/o Breadcrumbs
0.0	0.5	pc	SANDWICH, Ham Salad, Whole Wheat
0.0	75	g	SQUID, Fried
0.0	125	g	CHICKEN À LA KING
0.0	100	g	LAMB, Neck Fillet, Lean Only
0.0	1	pc	CHICKEN THIGH, w/Skin, Fried, Batter
0.0	250	g	SOUP, Cream of Chicken
0.0	75	g	GOOSE, Meat and Skin, Baked
0.0	50	g	SAUSAGE, Polish
0.0	100	g	SALMON TROUT, Scotch Smoked
0.0	150	g	SHEPHERD'S PIE, Frozen, Tesco's
0.0	50	g	SALAMI, Beef
0.0	2	pc	CHICKEN WING, w/Skin, Baked
−0.5	75	g	BEEF TONGUE, Simmered
−0.5	75	g	VEAL CHOP, Med. Fat, Fried
−0.5	100	g	CORNED BEEF, Sainsbury's Premium
−0.5	100	g	HASH

Nutripoints	Serving Size		Food Name
−0.5	50	g	PORK CHOP, Grilled
−0.5	2	pc	MEATBALLS
−0.5	1	pc	CHICKEN WING, w/Skin, Fried, Batter
−0.5	75	g	LOBSTER, Floured/Breaded, Fried
−0.5	75	g	MEATLOAF
−0.5	75	g	BEEF T-BONE STEAK, Med. Fat, Grilled
−0.5	50	g	SAUSAGE, Italian
−0.5	250	g	SOUP, Clam Chowder
−0.5	75	g	COD, Floured/Breaded, Fried
−0.5	0.5	pc	SANDWICH, Ham Salad, White
−0.5	75	g	PLAICE, Fillet, Breaded, Fried
−0.5	150	g	CHOW MEIN, Tesco's
−0.5	75	g	CARP, Floured/Breaded, Fried
−0.5	50	g	LAMB CHOP, Loin, Med. Fat, Baked
−0.5	100	g	LAMB, Roast Shoulder, Lean Only
−1.0	1	pc	PORK CHOP, Pan-Fried
−1.0	75	g	HADDOCK, Floured/Breaded, Fried
−1.0	75	g	PORK, Loin Chop, Grilled, Lean and Fat
−1.0	250	g	SOUP, Chicken & Veg, Campbell's
−1.0	75	g	DUCK, Meat and Skin, Baked
−1.0	75	g	LAMB SHOULDER, Med. Fat, Baked
−1.0	100	g	LOBSTER, Baked/Grilled with Butter
−1.0	25	g	PATÉ, de Foie Gras, Canned (Goose Liver)
−1.0	3	pc	SCAMPI
−1.0	50	g	BEEF SHORT RIBS, Med. Fat, Braised
−1.0	100	g	COD STEAK/CRISPY BATTER, Baked, Tesco's
−1.0	100	g	CRAB SALAD
−1.0	1	pc	FRANKFURTER, Chicken, with Bun
−1.0	50	g	BRATWURST
−1.0	75	g	CRAB, Soft Shell, Fried
−1.0	1	pc	KENTUCKY FRIED CHICKEN
−1.0	3	pc	BACON, Fried
−1.5	50	g	SPAM

Nutripoints	Serving Size		Food Name
−1.5	3	pc	PORK SPARERIBS
−1.5	0.5	pc	VEAL PARMIGIANI
−1.5	75	g	BACON RASHERS, Rindless, Sainsbury's
−1.5	75	g	BACON CHOPS, Tendersweet, Sainsbury's
−1.5	150	g	SKATE WING, Fried in Batter
−1.5	75	g	HALIBUT, Smoked
−1.5	175	g	SQUID, Boiled
−2.0	2	pc	FROGS' LEGS, Fried
−2.0	50	g	BEEF SIRLOIN STEAK, Grilled
−2.0	75	g	BEEFBURGER, Frozen, Tesco's
−2.0	50	g	PORK CHIPOLATAS, Tesco's
−2.0	100	g	KEDGEREE (with Smoked Fish, Rice & Egg)
−2.0	50	g	BACON, Back, Grilled, Sainsbury's Premium
−2.5	50	g	SAMOSA, Meat-Filled
−2.5	50	g	BACON, Streaky, Sainsbury's Grilled
−2.5	1	pc	FRANKFURTER, Beef
−2.5	50	g	BEEF PRIME RIB, Baked
−2.5	50	g	PASTRAMI, Beef
−2.5	50	g	SAUSAGE, Pork, Wall's Best English
−2.5	75	g	CORNED BEEF
−3.0	75	g	FRANKFURTERS, German, Sainsbury's Original
−3.0	50	g	LUNCHEON MEAT, Pork, Prince's
−3.0	100	g	LAMB/Hot Onion & Tom Sce, Bhuna Gosht, Sainsbury's
−3.5	50	g	BOLOGNA, Beef
−3.5	50	g	SALAMI, Black Peppered, Tesco's
−3.5	250	g	SOUP, Crm of Chicken, Spec. Rec., Heinz
−3.5	1	pc	FRANKFURTER, Pork & Beef
−3.5	100	g	LAMB KIDNEY, Fried
−4.0	250	g	SOUP, Chicken & Mushroom, Heinz
−4.0	25	g	SALT PORK, Raw
−5.0	25	g	PEPPERONI
−52.0	75	g	SWEETBREADS

Top-Ten Nutripoint Foods

For easy reference, the following lists are a handy breakdown of the top-ten foods in each of the Nutrigroups.

Vegetables	*Fruits*
Turnip tops	Cantaloupe melon
Spinach	Guava
Bok choy	Papaya
Parsley	Strawberries
Broccoli	Blackcurrants
Watercress	Mango
Asparagus	Kiwi fruit
Red peppers	Litchi
Swiss chard	Mandarin oranges
Canned tomatoes	Honeydew melon

*Grains**	*Pulses/Nuts/Seeds*
Wheat bran	Bean sprouts
Wheat germ	Frozen peas
High fibre Ryvita snackbread	Green peas
Bemax	Green mung beans
Weetabix	Black-eyed peas
Whole wheat muffin	Kidney beans
Wholemeal flour	French beans
Wholemeal bread	Split lentils
Quaker puffed wheat cereal	Split peas
Shredded wheat cereal	Garbanzo beans

Milk/Dairy	*Meat/Fish/Poultry*
Vital skimmed milk	Raw clams
Skimmed milk powder	Raw oysters
Build up	Calf's liver
Very low fat yogurt	Baked venison
Skimmed milk soft cheese	Canned clams
Very low fat fromage frais	Tuna canned in water
Cultured buttermilk	Baked pike
Complan	Steamed salmon
Very low fat yogurt drink	Baked halibut
Egg white	Lamb's liver

* This list excludes fortified cereals

NUTRIPOINT FOOD RATINGS
Fat/Oil Group

Nutripoints	Serving Size		Food Name
4.5	125	ml	SAUCE, White, Packet Mix Made w/Skim Milk
3.0	2	T	SAUCE, Bread, Homemade with Skim Milk
1.5	50	ml	SAUCE MIX, Stroganoff, made w/Milk & Water
1.0	50	ml	SAUCE MIX, Mushroom, made w/Milk
1.0	50	ml	GRAVY, Beef, Canned
0.5	100	ml	SAUCE, Cheese, Packet Mix made w/Skim Milk
0.0	50	ml	GRAVY MIX, Chicken, Prepared
0.0	50	ml	SAUCE MIX, Curry, made with Milk
0.0	50	ml	SAUCE MIX, Sweet and Sour, Prepared
−0.5	1	T	SAUCE, Tartare, Kraft
−0.5	50	ml	GRAVY MIX, Turkey, Prepared
−0.5	50	ml	GRAVY MIX, Mushroom, Prepared
−1.0	50	ml	SAUCE, White
−1.0	2	T	DRESSING, Salad, Low Cal
−1.5	2	T	DRESSING, Low Cal, French
−1.5	50	g	SPREAD, Very Low Fat, Outline
−1.5	50	g	SPREAD, Very Low Fat, Gold Lowest
−2.0	50	ml	GRAVY MIX, Pork, Prepared
−2.0	30	g	SPREAD, Sunflower, Low Fat, Flora Ex. Light
−2.5	30	g	SPREAD, Low Fat, Unsalted, Gold
−2.5	30	g	SPREAD, Mello, Kraft
−2.5	30	g	SPREAD, Sunflower, Red. Fat, Vitalite Light
−2.5	1	T	OIL, Rapeseed, Sainsbury's
−2.5	2	T	DRESSING, Russian
−2.5	30	g	SPREAD, Low Fat, Gold
−2.5	1	T	OIL, Hazelnut
−2.5	1	T	OIL, Blended Vegetable, Spry Crisp 'n' Dry
−2.5	1	T	OIL, Blended Vegetable, Sainsbury's

Nutripoints	Serving Size		Food Name
−2.5	1	T	OIL, Almond
−2.5	4	T	SALAD CREAM, Average, Reduced Calorie
−2.5	1	T	OIL, Vegetable
−2.5	1	T	OIL, Walnut
−2.5	1	T	OIL, Walnut, Sainsbury's
−2.5	1	T	OIL, Safflower
−2.5	1	T	OIL, Linseed
−2.5	15	g	SUET, Shredded Beef, Copperfields
−2.5	15	g	SPREAD, Red. Fat, Slightly Salted, Clover
−2.5	15	g	SPREAD, Reduced Fat, Clover
−2.5	15	g	MARGARINE, Corn Oil
−2.5	1	T	OIL, Sunflower, Flora
−2.5	2	T	MAYONNAISE, Low Cal
−2.5	1	T	OIL, Grapeseed, Sainsbury's
−2.5	30	g	SPREAD, Low Fat, Delight
−2.5	1	T	OIL, Sunflower
−2.5	15	g	MARGARINE, Hard
−2.5	50	ml	GRAVY MIX, Turkey, made w/Milk & Butter
−2.5	50	ml	GRAVY
−2.5	50	ml	GRAVY MIX, Chicken, made w/Milk & Butter
−2.5	15	g	MARGARINE, Sunflower, Flora
−2.5	2	T	DRESSING, Italian
−2.5	2	T	MAYONNAISE, Light Reduced Calorie, Kraft
−2.5	15	g	MARGARINE, Soft, Sainsbury's
−2.5	15	g	MARGARINE, Sunflower, Blue Band
−2.5	1	T	MAYONNAISE
−3.0	2	T	DRESSING, Thousand Island
−3.0	1	T	OIL, Soybean
−3.0	2	T	MAYONNAISE, Light Reduced Cal, Hellman's
−3.0	15	g	MARGARINE
−3.0	1	T	OIL, Olive, Sainsbury's
−3.0	1	T	OIL, Olive

Nutripoints	Serving Size		Food Name
−3.0	1	T	OIL, Corn, Mazola
−3.0	1	T	OIL, Sesame
−3.0	1	T	OIL, Soya, Sainsbury's
−3.0	1	T	OIL, Olive, Bertolli
−3.0	15	g	MARGARINE, Soya, Sainsbury's
−3.0	1	T	OIL, Sesame Seed, Dufrais
−3.0	1	T	OIL, Peanut
−3.0	1	T	OIL, Hazelnut, Sainsbury's
−3.0	1	T	DRESSING, Oil & Vinegar
−3.0	2	T	DRESSING, French
−3.0	1	T	DRESSING, French, Home Recipe
−3.0	15	g	SHORTENING, Polyunsaturated, White Flora
−3.0	1	T	OIL, Wheat Germ
−3.0	2	T	DRESSING, Blue Cheese
−3.5	1	T	MAYONNAISE, Average
−3.5	2	T	SAUCE, Tartare
−3.5	1	T	MAYONNAISE, Homemade with Olive Oil
−3.5	1	T	MAYONNAISE, Real, Hellman's
−3.5	1	T	OIL, Cottonseed
−3.5	15	g	SPREAD, Golden Churn, Kraft
−3.5	15	g	SHORTENING, Vegetable, Trex
−3.5	15	g	MARGARINE, Luxury Soft, Sainsbury's
−3.5	30	g	SPREAD, Low Fat, Clover Light
−4.0	15	g	GHEE, Vegetable, Sharwood's
−4.0	15	g	OIL, Solid Vegetable, Spry Crisp 'n' Dry
−4.0	1	T	FAT, Goose
−4.5	1	T	FAT, Chicken
−4.5	15	g	SPREAD, Dairy Master, Golden Churn
−4.5	1	T	FAT, Turkey
−4.5	1	T	FAT, Duck
−5.0	15	g	SPREAD, Willow
−5.0	15	g	SPREAD, Krona Spreadable

Nutripoints	Serving Size		Food Name
−5.0	1	T	OIL, Palm
−5.0	15	g	LARD
−5.0	4	T	SAUCE, Hollandaise
−5.5	4	T	SAUCE MIX, Bearnaise, Made w/Milk-Butter
−5.5	15	g	BUTTER, Lurpak, Unsalted
−5.5	1	T	OIL, Cocoa Butter
−5.5	15	g	SPREAD, Summer County
−5.5	15	g	SPREAD, Krona
−6.0	30	g	SPREAD, Half Fat, Anchor
−6.5	15	g	MARGARINE, Stork Special Blend
−6.5	15	g	SPREAD, Reduced Fat, Stork Light Blend
−6.5	15	g	BUTTER, Eng. Unsalt., Continental Taste, Sains.
−6.5	1	T	OIL, Palm Kernel
−7.0	15	g	BUTTER, Unsalted, Lurpak
−7.0	15	g	BUTTER, Concentrated, Buttacook
−7.0	15	g	BUTTER, Slightly Salted, Sweetcream
−7.0	15	g	MARGARINE, Echo
−7.0	1	T	OIL, Coconut
−7.5	15	g	FAT, Refined Cooking, Cookeen
−7.5	15	g	BUTTER, Salted
−7.5	15	g	FAT, Refined Cooking, White Cap

Sugar Group

Nutripoints	Serving Size		Food Name
−1.0	4	T	JAM, Low Cal, All Flavours
−1.0	6	pc	GINGER SNAPS
−1.5	30	g	CHOCOLATE, Cadbury's Dairy Milk
−1.5	30	g	CHOCOLATE, Cadbury's Bourneville
−2.0	25	g	HALVA, Plain
−2.0	25	g	CHOCOLATE, M and M's, Peanut
−2.0	1	pc	KIT KAT BAR, Rowntree's
−3.0	10	pc	GUMS, Fruit, Rowntree's
−3.0	2	T	MOLASSES
−3.5	1	pc	MILK CHOC BAR, with Almonds
−3.5	0.5	pc	MARS BAR
−3.5	2	T	SAUCE, Chocolate Fudge
−4.0	2	pc	MARS Twix
−4.0	1	pc	FUDGE, Vanilla
−4.0	0.5	pc	MILKY WAY
−4.0	25	g	CHOCOLATE, Baking
−4.5	40	g	NESTLÉ CHOCOLATE DAIRY CRUNCH
−4.5	3	T	ICING SUGAR
−4.5	5	pc	ROLOS
−4.5	10	pc	GUM, Doublemint, Wrigley's
−4.5	2	T	SAUCE, Butterscotch
−5.0	2	T	SYRUP, Maple
−5.0	2	T	MARMALADE
−5.0	2	T	SUGAR, Brown
−5.0	2	T	SAUCE, Chocolate
−5.0	2	T	SUGAR, Raw
−5.0	325	ml	SOFT DRINK, Ginger Ale

Nutripoints	Serving Size		Food Name
−5.5	25	g	FUDGE, Chocolate
−5.5	50	g	MOUSSE, Chocolate
−5.5	4	pc	MARSHMALLOWS
−5.5	30	g	TOFFEE ASSORTMENT, Sainsbury's
−5.5	2	T	HONEY
−5.5	325	ml	TONIC WATER, Sweetened
−5.5	325	ml	SOFT DRINK, 7-Up
−5.5	325	ml	SOFT DRINK, Cream Soda
−5.5	15	pc	JELLY BEANS
−6.0	5	pc	GUM, Bubble
−6.0	2	T	SUGAR, White
−6.0	325	ml	SOFT DRINK, Coke

Alcohol Group

Nutripoints	Serving Size		Food Name
1.0	325	ml	BEER, Non-Alcoholic
−7.5	75	ml	PINA COLADA
−8.0	325	ml	BEER
−8.5	325	ml	STOUT
−8.5	50	ml	ADVOCAT
−9.5	225	ml	SCREWDRIVER
−10.0	325	ml	BEER, Bitter
−10.0	150	ml	TEQUILA SUNRISE
−10.5	150	ml	RUM AND CARBONATED BEVERAGE
−10.5	325	ml	BEER, Lager
−11.0	150	ml	BLOODY MARY
−11.0	225	ml	GIN AND TONIC
−11.5	75	ml	VERMOUTH, Sweet
−11.5	50	ml	MAI TAI
−12.0	75	ml	ALEXANDER, Brandy
−12.5	75	ml	PORT
−12.5	50	ml	STINGER
−12.5	75	ml	RUM, Hot Buttered
−13.0	50	ml	BLACK RUSSIAN
−13.0	100	ml	WINE, White, Sweet
−13.0	50	ml	WHITE RUSSIAN
−13.0	50	ml	BACARDI
−13.0	50	ml	CURACAO
−13.5	150	ml	SINGAPORE SLING
−13.5	75	ml	MANHATTAN
−13.5	75	ml	MARGARITA
−14.0	100	ml	SHERRY, Sweet
−14.0	100	ml	WINE, White, Dry

Nutripoints	Serving Size		Food Name
−14.0	225	ml	TOM COLLINS
−14.0	100	ml	VERMOUTH, Dry
−14.5	150	ml	WINE SPRITZER
−14.5	75	ml	DAIQUIRI
−15.0	100	ml	CHAMPAGNE
−15.0	50	ml	MINT JULEP
−15.5	100	ml	WINE, Red
−15.5	50	ml	OLD FASHIONED
−15.5	150	ml	GIN RICKEY
−15.5	75	ml	MARTINI
−15.5	100	ml	SHERRY, Dry
−16.5	50	ml	WHISKY
−16.5	50	ml	VODKA
−16.5	50	ml	RUM
−17.0	150	ml	BOURBON OR SCOTCH WITH SODA
−17.0	75	ml	BRANDY
−17.5	50	ml	GIN
−19.0	75	ml	WHISKY SOUR

Condiment Group

Nutripoints	Serving Size		Food Name
2.5	1	T	PEPPERS, Green, Hot Chilli
2.5	0.25	pc	LEMON
2.5	1	tsp	PAPRIKA
2.0	1	tsp	CHILLI POWDER
1.5	1	tsp	PEPPER, Cayenne/Red
1.0	2	pc	ONION, Spring
1.0	1	T	CHIVES, Raw
1.0	1	tsp	SAUCE, Worcestershire
1.0	1	tsp	CINNAMON
1.0	1	tsp	OREGANO
1.0	1	T	SAUCE, Chilli
1.0	0.25	pc	ENDIVE, Raw
1.0	1	T	JUICE, Lemon
1.0	0.25	pc	LIME
1.0	20	g	ANCHOVIES, Canned
1.0	8	g	CORIANDER, Fresh
0.5	1	tsp	MARJORAM
0.5	1	tsp	CELERY SEED
0.5	1	tsp	BASIL
0.5	1	tsp	CHICKEN SEASONING
0.5	1	tsp	TURMERIC
0.5	1	tsp	GARLIC POWDER
0.5	1	tsp	THYME
0.5	1	tsp	CURRY POWDER
0.5	1	tsp	POPPY SEED
0.5	1	tsp	GINGER
0.5	1	tsp	DILL WEED
0.5	1	tsp	PEPPER, Black
0.5	1	tsp	CARAWAY SEED

Nutripoints	Serving Size		Food Name
0.5	1	tsp	SAGE
0.5	1	T	JUICE, Lime
0.5	1	tsp	BAY LEAVES
0.5	1	tsp	CLOVES
0.5	1	tsp	TARRAGON
0.5	1	tsp	ROSEMARY
0.5	1	tsp	PARSLEY, Dried
0.5	1	tsp	MUSTARD POWDER
0.5	1	tsp	ONION POWDER
0.5	1	tsp	ALLSPICE, Ground
0.5	1	pc	GARLIC, Raw
0.0	1	T	SAUCE, Barbeque
0.0	250	g	BROTH, Beef, Heinz Farmhouse
0.0	1	T	VINEGAR
0.0	250	g	BROTH, Beef
0.0	1	tsp	VANILLA EXTRACT
0.0	1	T	PICCALILLI
0.0	1	tsp	SALT
0.0	1	tsp	MUSTARD
0.0	1	tsp	SALT, Lo
0.0	250	g	BROTH, Chicken
0.0	1	T	HORSERADISH
0.0	1	tsp	NUTMEG
0.0	1	tsp	SAUCE, Soy
−1.5	1	T	SAUCE, Sweet and Sour
−2.0	225	g	BOUILLON CUBE, Chicken Flavour
−2.0	225	g	BOUILLON CUBE, Beef Flavour

Miscellaneous Group

Nutripoints	Serving Size		Food Name
3.5	1	T	YEAST, Brewers
2.0	1	T	GELATINE, Powdered
1.0	225	ml	LEMONADE, Low Calorie, Sainsbury's
1.0	1	T	CAROB POWDER
0.5	225	ml	COFFEE, Decaffeinated
0.5	1	tsp	BAKING POWDER
0.5	150	ml	TEA, Herb
0.5	250	g	CONSOMMÉ
0.5	1	T	COCOA POWDER
0.0	225	ml	TEA, Decaffeinated
0.0	8	g	YEAST, Dry Active
0.0	1	T	CORNFLOWER
0.0	225	ml	PERRIER MINERAL WATER
0.0	150	ml	CLUB SODA
-3.0	225	ml	TEA, Infused
-3.5	225	ml	COFFEE, Fresh
-10.0	1	tsp	COFFEE, Instant
-11.5	1	T	CAVIAR

Food Name Report

Name	Group	Serving Size		Points
ABALONE	Meat/Fish/Poultry	75	g	6.5
Floured, Fried	Meat/Fish/Poultry	75	g	4.5
ADVOCAT	Alcohol	50	ml	−8.5
ALEXANDER, Brandy	Alcohol	75	ml	−12.0
ALFALFA SPROUTS, Raw	Vegetable	75	g	17.5
ALLSPICE, Ground	Condiment	1	tsp	0.5
ALMOND BUTTER, Salted	Pulse/Nut/Seed	1	T	0.5
ALMOND KERNELS	Pulse/Nut/Seed	18	pc	1.5
ALMONDS, Chocolate-Covered	Pulse/Nut/Seed	6	pc	−1.0
Oil Roasted, Salted	Pulse/Nut/Seed	12	pc	0.5
Sugar-Coated	Pulse/Nut/Seed	6	pc	−1.5
ANCHOVY, Canned	Condiment	20	g	1.0
ANGEL DELIGHT,				
Sugar Free, Bird's	Milk/Dairy	100	g	3.5
Sugar Free, Wild Strawberry	Milk/Dairy	100	g	0.0
APPLE, Fresh	Fruit	1	pc	4.5
Stewed, with Sugar	Fruit	125	g	−0.5
APRICOT NECTAR, Canned	Fruit	100	ml	4.5
APRICOTS,				
Canned, Heavy Syrup	Fruit	125	g	2.5
Canned, Unsweetened	Fruit	125	g	11.0
Dried	Fruit	6	pc	11.0
Dried, Whitworths	Fruit	6	pc	11.5
Fresh	Fruit	3	pc	13.5
ARTICHOKE, Cooked	Vegetable	1	pc	12.5
ARTICHOKE HEARTS,				
Marinated	Vegetable	60	g	3.0
ASPARAGUS, Canned	Vegetable	8	pc	32.5
Cuts, Canned, Green Giant	Vegetable	125	g	14.0

Name	Group	Serving Size		Points
Fresh	Vegetable	8	pc	44.0
Frozen, Boiled	Vegetable	8	pc	27.0
AUBERGINE, Cooked	Vegetable	100	g	17.0
AVOCADO, California	Fruit	0.25	pc	2.5
Florida	Fruit	0.25	pc	4.0
BACARDI	Alcohol	50	ml	−13.0
BACON,				
Back, Grilled, Sains. Premium	Meat/Fish/Poultry	50	g	−2.0
Danish	Meat/Fish/Poultry	3	pc	1.5
Fried	Meat/Fish/Poultry	3	pc	−1.0
Streaky, Sainsbury's Grilled	Meat/Fish/Poultry	50	g	−2.5
BACON CHOPS,				
Tendersweet, Sainsbury's	Meat/Fish/Poultry	75	g	−1.5
BACON RASHERS,				
Rindless Dutch, Sains.	Meat/Fish/Poultry	75	g	−1.5
BAGEL	Grain	1	pc	2.0
BAKING POWDER	Miscellaneous	1	tsp	0.5
BAMBOO SHOOTS, Canned	Vegetable	125	g	16.5
Raw	Vegetable	75	g	17.0
BANANA	Fruit	0.5	pc	7.5
BANANA SPLIT	Fruit	0.25	pc	−1.5
BARRACUDA, Baked/Grilled	Meat/Fish/Poultry	75	g	1.5
Breaded/Floured, Fried	Meat/Fish/Poultry	75	g	1.0
BASIL	Condiment	1	tsp	0.5
BASS, Freshwater, Baked	Meat/Fish/Poultry	175	g	7.0
BAY LEAVES	Condiment	1	tsp	0.5
BEAN SPROUTS, Mung, Fresh	Pulse/Nut/Seed	200	g	18.0
BEAN, Mung, Green	Pulse/Nut/Seed	200	g	10.5
BEANS,				
Baked, in Tomato Sauce, Heinz	Pulse/Nut/Seed	150	g	5.5
Baked, in Tomato Sauce, Top Crop	Pulse/Nut/Seed	220	g	6.5

Name	Group	Serving Size		Points
Baked, in Tomato Sauce	Pulse/Nut/Seed	125	g	7.5
Boston Baked	Pulse/Nut/Seed	125	g	3.5
French, Boiled	Pulse/Nut/Seed	150	g	8.5
Garbanzo, Cooked	Pulse/Nut/Seed	75	g	8.0
Green, Cut, Frozen, Bird's Eye	Vegetable	100	g	15.5
Green, Whole, Canned	Vegetable	200	g	13.0
Kidney, Red	Pulse/Nut/Seed	125	g	8.5
Pinto, Cooked	Pulse/Nut/Seed	125	g	6.5
With Pork	Pulse/Nut/Seed	125	g	3.0
BEEF BRISKET, Lean, Braised	Meat/Fish/Poultry	75	g	2.0
BEEF CHUCK ROAST,				
Lean, Braised	Meat/Fish/Poultry	75	g	3.5
Med. Fat, Baked	Meat/Fish/Poultry	50	g	0.5
BEEF FLANK STEAK,				
Lean, Grilled	Meat/Fish/Poultry	75	g	4.0
Med. Fat, Choice, Grilled	Meat/Fish/Poultry	75	g	1.5
BEEF HEART, Braised	Meat/Fish/Poultry	75	g	4.0
BEEF LIVER, Fried	Meat/Fish/Poultry	75	g	7.0
BEEF PASTE, Tesco's	Meat/Fish/Poultry	75	g	1.0
BEEF PORTERHOUSE STEAK,				
Lean, Grilled	Meat/Fish/Poultry	75	g	2.5
BEEF POT PIE	Meat/Fish/Poultry	0.5	pc	0.5
BEEF PRIME RIB, Baked	Meat/Fish/Poultry	50	g	−2.5
BEEF RIB EYE, Lean, Grilled	Meat/Fish/Poultry	75	g	2.5
BEEF RIBS, Baked	Meat/Fish/Poultry	75	g	2.0
BEEF ROUND STEAK,				
Lean, Grilled	Meat/Fish/Poultry	75	g	4.0
Med. Fat, Grilled	Meat/Fish/Poultry	75	g	2.0
BEEF RUMP ROAST, Baked	Meat/Fish/Poultry	50	g	0.5
BEEF SHORT RIBS,				
Lean, Braised	Meat/Fish/Poultry	75	g	1.0
Med. Fat, Braised	Meat/Fish/Poultry	50	g	−1.0

Name	Group	Serving Size		Points
BEEF SIRLOIN STEAK, Grilled	Meat/Fish/Poultry	50	g	−2.0
BEEF SIRLOIN, Roast Lean	Meat/Fish/Poultry	100	g	2.5
BEEF STEW	Meat/Fish/Poultry	250	g	3.5
BEEF STROGANOFF	Meat/Fish/Poultry	125	g	0.0
BEEF T-BONE STEAK,				
Lean, Choice, Grilled	Meat/Fish/Poultry	75	g	2.5
Med. Fat, Grilled	Meat/Fish/Poultry	75	g	−0.5
BEEF TENDERLOIN FILLET,				
Lean, Grilled	Meat/Fish/Poultry	75	g	3.5
Med. Fat, Grilled	Meat/Fish/Poultry	75	g	1.0
BEEF TONGUE, Simmered	Meat/Fish/Poultry	75	g	−0.5
BEEF TOP LOIN, Lean, Grilled	Meat/Fish/Poultry	75	g	4.0
Med. Fat, Grilled	Meat/Fish/Poultry	75	g	0.5
BEEF TOPSIDE, Roast Lean	Meat/Fish/Poultry	100	g	4.0
BEEF, Macaroni and				
Tomato Sauce	Meat/Fish/Poultry	175	g	3.0
BEEFBURGER, Frozen, Tesco's	Meat/Fish/Poultry	75	g	−2.0
BEER	Alcohol	325	ml	−8.0
Bitter	Alcohol	325	ml	−10.0
Lager	Alcohol	325	ml	−10.5
Non-alcoholic	Alcohol	325	ml	1.0
BEMAX	Grain	40	g	8.0
BISCUITS, Chocolate	Grain	30	g	−2.0
BISCUITS, Plain Digestives	Grain	30	g	−2.0
BLACK RUSSIAN	Alcohol	50	ml	−13.0
BLACKBERRIES, Fresh	Fruit	75	g	13.0
Frozen, Unsweetened	Fruit	75	g	7.5
BLOODY MARY	Alcohol	150	ml	−11.0
BLUEBERRIES, Fresh	Fruit	75	g	7.0
BOK CHOY, Raw, Shredded	Vegetable	150	g	72.5
BOLOGNA, Beef	Meat/Fish/Poultry	50	g	−3.5
BOLOGNESE,				
Spaghetti, Chilled, Tesco's	Meat/Fish/Poultry	150	g	2.0

Name	Group	Serving Size		Points
BOUILLON CUBE, Beef Flavour	Condiment	125	g	−2.0
Chicken Flavour	Condiment	225	g	−2.0
BOURBON OR SCOTCH w/Soda	Alcohol	150	ml	−17.0
BRAN, Wheat	Grain	25	g	26.5
BRANDY	Alcohol	75	ml	−17.0
BRATWURST	Meat/Fish/Poultry	50	g	−1.0
BRAZIL NUT KERNELS	Pulse/Nut/Seed	6	pc	0.0
BREAD, Banana	Grain	1	pc	−0.5
Cracked Wheat	Grain	2	pc	4.5
French	Grain	2	pc	3.0
Garlic	Grain	1	pc	0.0
Hi-fibre, Vitbe	Grain	3	pc	3.5
Italian	Grain	2	pc	2.5
Mix Grain, Mighty White	Grain	3	pc	4.0
Nimble	Grain	14	pc	2.5
Pitta	Grain	1	pc	3.5
Pitta, Whole Wheat	Grain	1	pc	4.0
Pumpernickel	Grain	2	pc	4.5
Rye, Light	Grain	2	pc	3.0
Soda	Grain	1	pc	2.5
Wheat Germ	Grain	2	pc	4.0
Wheat, Stone Ground	Grain	2	pc	3.5
White	Grain	2	pc	2.5
White Fried	Grain	1	pc	−3.5
White, Toasted	Grain	3	pc	2.0
Whole Meal	Grain	2	pc	6.0
Whole Rye	Grain	2	pc	4.0
BREAD & BUTTER PUDDING	Grain	100	g	−4.0
BREADCRUMBS	Grain	40	g	2.0
BREAD ROLL, White, Crusty	Grain	1	pc	2.5
BREADSTICKS	Grain	6	pc	3.5
Garlic	Grain	6	pc	1.0

Name	Group	Serving Size		Points
BROCCOLI SPEARS,				
Frozen, Bird's Eye	Vegetable	100	g	46.0
BROCCOLI,				
Caul & Crts, Cheese Sauce	Vegetable	100	g	13.0
Caul & Rd Pprs, Fz, Bird's Eye	Vegetable	125	g	41.5
Cooked	Vegetable	175	g	38.5
Corn & Red Pprs, Fz, Bird's Eye	Vegetable	125	g	17.0
Raw	Vegetable	100	g	53.0
BROTH, Beef	Condiment	250	g	0.0
Beef, Heinz Farmhouse	Condiment	250	g	0.0
Chicken	Condiment	250	g	0.0
BRUSSELS SPROUTS, Cooked	Vegetable	75	g	40.0
Frozen, Cooked	Vegetable	75	g	27.0
BUILD UP,				
Made w/Skimmed Milk	Milk/Dairy	150	ml	15.0
Made w/Whole Milk	Milk/Dairy	100	ml	8.5
BULGAR, Dry	Grain	40	g	3.0
BUN, Hot Dog	Grain	1	pc	1.5
Submarine	Grain	0.5	pc	3.0
White Hamburger	Grain	1	pc	2.0
BURGER KING				
VANILLA SHAKE	Milk/Dairy	0.5	pc	−2.5
BUTTER,				
Concentrated, Buttacook	Fat/Oil	15	g	−7.0
Eng. Unsalt., Continental				
Taste, Sains.	Fat/Oil	15	g	−6.5
Lurpak, Unsalted	Fat/Oil	15	g	−5.5
Salted	Fat/Oil	15	g	−7.5
Slightly Salted, Sweetcream	Fat/Oil	15	g	−7.0
Unsalted, Lurpak	Fat/Oil	15	g	−7.0
BUTTERMILK,				
Cultured, Eden Vale	Milk/Dairy	225	ml	7.5

Name	Group	Serving Size		Points
Fresh	Milk/Dairy	225	ml	5.0
BUTTERNUTS	Pulse/Nut/Seed	25	g	1.0
CABBAGE,				
Common, Chopped, Cooked	Vegetable	175	g	31.5
Common, Raw, Shredded	Vegetable	100	g	39.0
Red, Raw, Shredded	Vegetable	75	g	29.5
Savoy, Raw, Shredded	Vegetable	75	g	24.5
CAKE, Cheese, w/Fruit Topping	Milk/Dairy	0.5	pc	−2.0
Coffee	Grain	0.5	pc	−2.0
Devil's Food	Grain	0.5	pc	−3.0
Dutch Apple	Grain	0.5	pc	−3.5
German Chocolate	Grain	0.5	pc	−3.0
Madeira	Grain	40	g	−2.5
Sponge, Fatless	Grain	30	g	−5.0
Sponge, Jam Filled	Grain	30	g	−3.5
Sponge, with Icing	Grain	0.5	pc	−3.5
CALF LIVER, Fried	Meat/Fish/Poultry	175	g	9.0
CANNELLONI,				
Cheese, Lean Cuisine	Milk/Dairy	0.5	pc	0.5
CAPON, Baked w/Skin	Meat/Fish/Poultry	75	g	1.5
CARAMBOLA (Starfruit)	Fruit	1	pc	12.5
CARAWAY SEED	Condiment	1	tsp	0.5
CAROB POWDER	Miscellaneous	1	T	1.0
CARP, Baked/Grilled	Meat/Fish/Poultry	75	g	0.5
Floured/Breaded, Fried	Meat/Fish/Poultry	75	g	−0.5
Smoked	Meat/Fish/Poultry	75	g	2.5
CARROTS, Raw	Vegetable	1	pc	35.5
Sliced, Cooked	Vegetable	75	g	30.0
CASHEW BUTTER, Salted	Pulse/Nut/Seed	25	g	0.5
CASHEWS, Dry Roasted, Salted	Pulse/Nut/Seed	25	g	0.5
Dry Roasted, Unsalted	Pulse/Nut/Seed	12	pc	1.5
Dry Roasted, Unsalt., Planter's	Pulse/Nut/Seed	25	g	1.5

Name	Group	Serving Size		Points
Oil Roasted, Salted	Pulse/Nut/Seed	25	g	0.5
Oil Roasted, Unsalted	Pulse/Nut/Seed	25	g	0.5
CAULIFLOWER, Cooked	Vegetable	125	g	37.5
Fried, w/Breadcrumbs	Vegetable	50	g	−0.5
Fz, Bird's Eye	Vegetable	175	g	23.0
Raw	Vegetable	100	g	40.5
CAULIFLOWER CHEESE,				
Marks & Spencer's	Vegetable	50	g	2.0
CAVIAR	Miscellaneous	1	T	−11.5
CELERIAC, Raw	Vegetable	75	g	8.0
CELERY SEED	Condiment	1	tsp	0.5
CELERY, Raw	Vegetable	8	pc	20.0
CEREAL,				
100% Bran w/Oat Bran,				
Nabisco	Grain	25	g	23.5
All Bran, Kellogg's	Grain	25	g	27.0
Alpen	Grain	25	g	3.5
Bran Buds, Kellogg's	Grain	50	g	14.0
Bran Flakes	Grain	30	g	14.5
Bran Flakes, Kellogg's	Grain	25	g	21.0
Clusters, Quaker	Grain	25	g	10.5
Coco Pops, Kellogg's	Grain	40	g	1.5
Corn Flakes, Kellogg's	Grain	25	g	18.0
Creusli, Alpen	Grain	40	g	4.0
Crunchy Nut Corn, Kellogg's	Grain	30	g	5.5
Frosties, Kellogg's	Grain	40	g	3.0
Grapenuts	Grain	40	g	14.5
Nutrigrain-Rye & Oats				
w/Hazel., Kellogg's	Grain	30	g	8.5
Oat Munchies, Quaker	Grain	25	g	17.0
Oatmeal, Raw	Grain	35	g	3.5
Porridge Oats, Quaker Scotts	Grain	100	g	2.0

Name	Group	Serving Size		Points
Puffed Rice	Grain	25	g	2.0
Puffed Wheat	Grain	25	g	4.5
Puffed Wheat, Quaker	Grain	25	g	5.5
Raisin Splitz, Kellogg's	Grain	25	g	14.0
Ready Brek, Lyons',				
Not Made Up	Grain	30	g	6.0
Rice Krispies, Kellogg's	Grain	25	g	11.5
Shredded Wheat, Nabisco	Grain	1	pc	5.0
Shredded Wheat, RHM	Grain	40	g	5.0
Shredded Wheat, Spoon Size	Grain	25	g	5.0
Special K, Kellogg's	Grain	25	g	14.0
Sultana Bran, Kellogg's	Grain	60	g	16.5
Team Flakes, RHM	Grain	25	g	11.5
Weetabix	Grain	40	g	6.5
Weetaflake, Weetabix	Grain	30	g	6.0
CEREAL BAR,				
Choc Chip Chewy, Jordon's	Grain	30	g	−2.0
CHAMPAGNE	Alcohol	100	ml	−15.0
CHEESE FONDUE	Milk/Dairy	4	T	−4.5
CHEESE SPREAD,				
Pasteurized Processed	Milk/Dairy	25	g	−3.0
Plain	Milk/Dairy	25	g	−1.5
CHEESE, Blue Stilton	Milk/Dairy	25	g	−3.0
Brie	Milk/Dairy	25	g	−2.0
Caerphilly	Milk/Dairy	25	g	−2.5
Camembert	Milk/Dairy	25	g	−1.0
Cheddar	Milk/Dairy	25	g	−2.0
Cheddar-type, Red. Fat,				
Tendale	Milk/Dairy	40	g	2.0
Cheshire	Milk/Dairy	25	g	−2.0
Cottage	Milk/Dairy	100	g	1.5
Cottage, Eden Vale Natural	Milk/Dairy	113	g	2.5

Name	Group	Serving Size		Points
Cottage, Half Fat, Sainsbury's	Milk/Dairy	125	g	4.0
Cottage, Low Fat, w/Pineapple	Milk/Dairy	125	g	1.5
Cottage, Very Low Fat, Shape	Milk/Dairy	150	g	5.5
Dairylea	Milk/Dairy	25	g	−3.0
Danish Blue	Milk/Dairy	25	g	−2.0
Double Gloucester	Milk/Dairy	25	g	−2.0
Edam	Milk/Dairy	25	g	−1.0
English Cheddar	Milk/Dairy	25	g	−2.0
Feta	Milk/Dairy	25	g	−2.5
Full Fat Soft, Philadelphia	Milk/Dairy	2	T	−5.5
Gouda	Milk/Dairy	25	g	−1.5
Grated, Parmesan	Milk/Dairy	25	g	0.5
Gruyère	Milk/Dairy	25	g	−1.0
Limburger	Milk/Dairy	25	g	−3.0
Mozzarella	Milk/Dairy	25	g	−1.5
Mozzarella, Low Fat	Milk/Dairy	25	g	0.5
Neufchatel	Milk/Dairy	25	g	−4.0
Provolone	Milk/Dairy	25	g	−1.0
Ricotta	Milk/Dairy	50	g	−2.0
Ricotta, Low Fat	Milk/Dairy	50	g	0.5
Romano	Milk/Dairy	25	g	−2.0
Roquefort	Milk/Dairy	25	g	−3.0
Skimmed Milk Soft, Quark	Milk/Dairy	150	g	9.5
Soft, Kraft Philadelphia	Milk/Dairy	2	T	−5.0
Swiss, Reduced Fat, Kraft	Milk/Dairy	25	g	0.5
White Stilton	Milk/Dairy	25	g	−3.0
CHEESECAKE,				
Frozen with Fruit Topping	Milk/Dairy	50	g	−3.0
CHERRIES,				
Cooking, Stewed, No Sugar	Fruit	125	g	11.5
Sour, Canned, Heavy Syrup	Fruit	125	g	1.0
Sour, Canned, Unsweetened	Fruit	125	g	7.5

Name	Group	Serving Size		Points
Sweet, Canned, Heavy Syrup	Fruit	125	g	0.0
Sweet, Fresh	Fruit	10	pc	5.5
CHERRY CHEESECAKE	Fruit	0.25	pc	−3.5
CHICKEN,				
Cornfed, Roast Meat Only	Meat/Fish/Poultry	100	g	0.5
Creamed	Meat/Fish/Poultry	125	g	1.5
CHICKEN À LA KING	Meat/Fish/Poultry	125	g	0.0
CHICKEN AND HAM PASTE,				
Tesco's	Meat/Fish/Poultry	25	g	1.0
CHICKEN BREAST,				
Baked w/o Skin	Meat/Fish/Poultry	75	g	4.0
Fried w/Batter, w/Skin	Meat/Fish/Poultry	75	g	1.0
Fried w/o Bread, w/Skin	Meat/Fish/Poultry	75	g	2.5
Fried w/o Skin	Meat/Fish/Poultry	75	g	1.5
CHICKEN FRICASSÉE	Meat/Fish/Poultry	125	g	2.5
CHICKEN FRIED STEAK	Meat/Fish/Poultry	50	g	0.0
CHICKEN GOUJONS, Tesco's	Meat/Fish/Poultry	100	g	0.5
CHICKEN KIEV	Meat/Fish/Poultry	0.5	pc	0.0
CHICKEN LEG, Baked w/o Skin	Meat/Fish/Poultry	75	g	2.5
Fried w/o Bread, w/Skin	Meat/Fish/Poultry	75	g	1.5
CHICKEN LIVER, Stewed	Meat/Fish/Poultry	75	g	2.0
CHICKEN POT PIE	Meat/Fish/Poultry	0.5	pc	0.5
CHICKEN SALAD	Meat/Fish/Poultry	100	g	2.0
CHICKEN SEASONING	Condiment	1	tsp	0.5
CHICKEN THIGH,				
Baked w/o Skin	Meat/Fish/Poultry	75	g	1.0
Fried w/o Breadcrumbs	Meat/Fish/Poultry	75	g	2.0
Meat & Skin, Baked	Meat/Fish/Poultry	1	pc	0.0
Meat & Skin, Fried, Batter	Meat/Fish/Poultry	1	pc	0.0
CHICKEN WING,				
Baked w/o Skin	Meat/Fish/Poultry	3	pc	2.0
Fried w/o Breadcrumbs	Meat/Fish/Poultry	2	pc	2.0

Name	Group	Serving Size		Points
Meat & Skin, Baked	Meat/Fish/Poultry	2	pc	0.0
Meat & Skin, Fried, Batter	Meat/Fish/Poultry	1	pc	−0.5
CHICKEN WITH DUMPLINGS	Meat/Fish/Poultry	150	g	2.0
CHICORY GREENS, Raw	Vegetable	175	g	35.5
CHILLI POWDER	Condiment	1	tsp	2.0
CHILLI w/LENTILS, Vegetarian	Pulse/Nut/Seed	125	g	3.0
CHILLI, Bean/Beef	Pulse/Nut/Seed	125	g	1.0
CHILLI, Beans	Pulse/Nut/Seed	100	g	5.0
CHIVES, Raw	Condiment	1	tsp	1.0
CHOCOLATE ECLAIR	Grain	0.5	pc	−2.0
CHOCOLATE, Baking	Sugar	25	g	−4.0
Cadbury's Bourneville	Sugar	30	g	−1.5
Cadbury's Dairy Milk	Sugar	30	g	−1.5
Hot	Milk/Dairy	225	ml	0.0
M and M's Peanut	Sugar	25	g	−2.0
Nestlé Dairy Crunch	Sugar	40	g	−4.5
CHOP SUEY, Beef/Pork	Meat/Fish/Poultry	125	g	0.5
CHOW MEIN, Tesco's	Meat/Fish/Poultry	150	g	−0.5
CINNAMON	Condiment	1	tsp	1.0
CLAMS, Breaded, Fried	Meat/Fish/Poultry	75	g	4.5
Canned	Meat/Fish/Poultry	150	g	8.0
Mixed Species, Raw	Meat/Fish/Poultry	175	g	13.5
Smoked, Canned in Oil	Meat/Fish/Poultry	75	g	5.0
Steamed/Boiled	Meat/Fish/Poultry	175	g	6.0
CLOVES	Condiment	1	tsp	0.5
CLUB SODA	Miscellaneous	150	ml	0.0
COCOA MIX,				
Hot, Sugar Free, Carnation	Milk/Dairy	450	ml	3.0
Sugar Free, Quik, Nestlé	Milk/Dairy	225	ml	2.5
COCOA POWDER	Miscellaneous	1	T	0.5
COCONUT	Fruit	1	T	−2.0
Bounty Bar	Fruit	1	pc	−3.5

Name	Group	Serving Size		Points
Raw	Fruit	25	g	−3.5
COD, Baked	Meat/Fish/Poultry	100	g	3.5
Baked Fillet	Meat/Fish/Poultry	150	g	4.5
Floured/Breaded, Fried	Meat/Fish/Poultry	75	g	−0.5
Smoked	Meat/Fish/Poultry	175	g	2.0
COD FILLET, Smoked, Poached	Meat/Fish/Poultry	150	g	3.0
Skinless, Sainsbury's Prime	Meat/Fish/Poultry	175	g	7.0
COD FISH FINGERS, Bird's Eye	Meat/Fish/Poultry	100	g	1.0
COD STEAK/CRISPY BATTER,				
Baked, Tesco's	Meat/Fish/Poultry	100	g	−1.0
COFFEE, Decaffeinated	Miscellaneous	225	ml	0.5
Fresh	Miscellaneous	225	ml	−3.5
Instant	Miscellaneous	1	tsp	−10.0
COLESLAW	Vegetable	50	g	3.0
COMPLAN,				
Savoury, made with Water	Milk/Dairy	100	ml	5.0
Sweet, made with Water	Milk/Dairy	100	ml	7.0
CONSOMMÉ	Miscellaneous	250	g	0.5
COOKIES, Chocolate Chip	Grain	2	pc	−4.0
Chocolate Chip Oatmeal	Grain	1	pc	−3.5
Filled Wafer	Grain	30	g	−3.0
French Vanilla Creme	Grain	2	pc	−1.5
Lemon Creme	Grain	4	pc	−1.5
Macaroon	Grain	2	pc	−2.0
Sandwich Biscuit	Grain	30	g	−2.5
CORIANDER, Fresh	Condiment	8	g	1.0
CORN CHIPS	Grain	25	g	−0.5
CORN MEAL, Dry	Grain	25	g	3.5
CORN ON COB, Fresh, Cooked	Vegetable	0.5	pc	6.0
CORN W/RED AND GREEN				
PEPPERS, Canned	Vegetable	125	g	5.0
CORN, Creamed, Canned	Vegetable	125	g	4.5

Name	Group	Serving Size		Points
Frozen, Cooked	Vegetable	75	g	8.0
Sweet, Frozen, Bird's Eye	Vegetable	100	g	6.0
Whole Kernel, Canned,				
Green Giant	Vegetable	125	g	2.5
CORNED BEEF	Meat/Fish/Poultry	75	g	−2.5
Sainsbury's Premium	Meat/Fish/Poultry	100	g	−0.5
CORNFLOUR	Miscellaneous	1	T	0.0
COURGETTES, Cooked	Vegetable	175	g	15.0
Raw	Vegetable	175	g	16.0
CRAB, Canned	Meat/Fish/Poultry	175	g	1.0
Hardshell, Steamed	Meat/Fish/Poultry	175	g	4.5
Soft Shell, Fried	Meat/Fish/Poultry	75	g	−1.0
CRAB SALAD	Meat/Fish/Poultry	100	g	−1.0
CRACKER,				
Crispbread Dark Rye, Ryvita	Grain	4	pc	3.0
Crispbread High Fibre	Grain	3	pc	7.5
Rice Cake	Grain	4	pc	1.5
Rice, Small	Grain	10	pc	0.5
Ritz	Grain	8	pc	−1.0
Snackbread, High Fibre, Ryvita	Grain	8	pc	9.0
Whole Wheat	Grain	8	pc	3.0
Cream	Grain	30	g	−1.5
Rye Crispbread	Grain	6	pc	5.0
Wheat Crispbread, Starch Red.	Grain	6	pc	3.0
CREAM, Double	Milk/Dairy	2	T	−7.0
Non-Dairy, Coffee Mate,				
Carnation	Milk/Dairy	2	T	−3.5
Non-Dairy, Imitation, Liquid				
(Veg. Oil)	Milk/Dairy	2	T	−1.5
Non-Dairy, Mocha Mix	Milk/Dairy	50	g	−2.0
Sour	Milk/Dairy	50	g	−3.5
Whipped	Milk/Dairy	4	T	−6.5

Name	Group	Serving Size		Points
CREME CARAMEL	Milk/Dairy	100	g	0.0
CRISPS	Vegetable	5	pc	0.0
CROISSANT	Grain	1	pc	−2.5
CUCUMBER, Raw	Vegetable	75	g	20.0
CUPCAKE, with Icing	Grain	1	pc	−4.0
Without Icing	Grain	1	pc	−3.5
CURACAO	Alcohol	50	ml	−13.0
CURRANTS, Black	Fruit	75	g	19.0
CURRY POWDER	Condiment	1	tsp	0.5
CUSTARD	Milk/Dairy	125	g	−4.0
Bird's, made with Whole Milk	Milk/Dairy	100	ml	0.0
Made with Skimmed Milk	Milk/Dairy	150	ml	4.0
DAIQUIRI	Alcohol	75	ml	−14.5
DANISH PASTRY	Grain	0.5	pc	−2.5
DATES	Fruit	5	pc	4.0
DILL WEED	Condiment	1	tsp	0.5
DIP, Bean	Pulse/Nut/Seed	2	T	3.5
DOUGHNUT	Grain	40	g	−3.0
Custard Filling	Grain	0.5	pc	−3.0
Jam	Grain	0.5	pc	−3.0
DRESSING, Blue Cheese	Fat/Oil	2	T	−3.0
French	Fat/Oil	2	T	−3.0
French, Home Recipe	Fat/Oil	1	T	−3.0
Italian	Fat/Oil	2	T	−2.5
Low Cal, French	Fat/Oil	2	T	−1.5
Oil & Vinegar	Fat/Oil	1	T	−3.0
Russian	Fat/Oil	2	T	−2.5
Salad, Low Cal	Fat/Oil	2	T	−1.0
Thousand Island	Fat/Oil	2	T	−3.0
Yogurt	Milk/Dairy	2	T	0.5
DRINKING CHOCOLATE,				
Made w/Skimmed Milk	Milk/Dairy	150	ml	3.5

Name	Group	Serving Size		Points
Made w/Whole Milk	Milk/Dairy	100	ml	−0.5
DUCK, Baked, without Skin	Meat/Fish/Poultry	75	g	1.5
Meat and Skin, Baked	Meat/Fish/Poultry	75	g	−1.0
ECLAIR, Chocolate	Grain	30	g	−4.5
EEL	Meat/Fish/Poultry	75	g	1.5
Smoked	Meat/Fish/Poultry	75	g	1.5
EGG, Boiled	Milk/Dairy	2	pc	−11.5
Devilled (1 pc = Whole Egg)	Milk/Dairy	1	pc	−10.5
Fried	Milk/Dairy	1	pc	−12.5
Hard Boiled	Milk/Dairy	2	pc	−11.5
Omelette,				
w/Ham/Cheese (1 pc = 3 Eggs)	Milk/Dairy	0.5	pc	−8.0
Poached	Milk/Dairy	2	pc	−11.5
Scrambled	Milk/Dairy	1	pc	−13.5
EGG McMUFFIN, McDonald's	Milk/Dairy	0.5	pc	−1.5
w/Sausage, McDonald's	Milk/Dairy	0.25	pc	−1.5
EGG NOODLES, Cooked	Grain	60	g	1.5
EGG SALAD	Milk/Dairy	75	g	−9.0
EGG WHITE	Milk/Dairy	6	pc	6.0
EGG YOLK	Milk/Dairy	2	pc	−15.0
EGGNOG	Milk/Dairy	125	g	−2.0
EGGS, Scotch	Milk/Dairy	100	g	−3.5
ENDIVE, Raw	Condiment	0.25	pc	1.0
FAT, Chicken	Fat/Oil	1	T	−4.5
Duck	Fat/Oil	1	T	−4.5
Goose	Fat/Oil	1	T	−4.0
Refined Cooking, Cookeen	Fat/Oil	15	g	−7.5
Refined Cooking, White Cap	Fat/Oil	15	g	−7.5
Turkey	Fat/Oil	1	T	−4.5
FETTUCINI, Cooked	Grain	75	g	1.0
FIGS, Dried	Fruit	2	pc	5.0
Fresh	Fruit	1	pc	4.0

Name	Group	Serving Size		Points
FISH, Fried	Meat/Fish/Poultry	75	g	0.5
Smoked	Meat/Fish/Poultry	75	g	3.5
FISH FINGERS	Meat/Fish/Poultry	4	pc	0.5
FLOUR, Plain White, Household	Grain	40	g	3.0
Potato	Vegetable	50	g	5.5
Soya, Full Fat	Grain	30	g	4.5
White	Grain	30	g	3.0
Wholemeal	Grain	40	g	6.0
FRANKFURTER, Beef	Meat/Fish/Poultry	1	pc	−2.5
Chicken, with Bun	Meat/Fish/Poultry	1	pc	−1.0
Pork & Beef	Meat/Fish/Poultry	1	pc	−3.5
FRANKFURTERS,				
German, Sains. Original	Meat/Fish/Poultry	75	g	−3.0
FRENCH FRIES	Vegetable	4	pc	1.0
FRENCH TOAST	Grain	1	pc	−2.5
FROGS' LEGS, Fried	Meat/Fish/Poultry	2	pc	−2.0
FROMAGE FRAIS, Plain	Milk/Dairy	100	g	1.0
Very Low Fat	Milk/Dairy	175	g	8.5
With Fruit, Sainsbury's	Milk/Dairy	60	g	−1.0
FRUIT COCKTAIL,				
Canned, Heavy Syrup	Fruit	125	g	1.0
Canned, Unsweetened	Fruit	225	g	10.0
FRUIT DRINK, Orange, Capri Sun	Fruit	150	ml	−5.5
FRUIT SALAD, Fresh	Fruit	100	g	13.0
FRUITCAKE, Plain	Grain	30	g	−2.0
FUDGE, Chocolate	Sugar	25	g	−5.5
Vanilla	Sugar	1	pc	−4.0
GARLIC, Raw	Condiment	1	pc	0.5
GARLIC POWDER	Condiment	1	tsp	0.5
GAZPACHO	Vegetable	250	g	1.5
GELATINE, Cherry Flavour	Fruit	125	g	−5.0
GHEE, Vegetable, Sharwood's	Fat/Oil	15	g	−4.0

Name	Group	Serving Size		Points
GIN	Alcohol	50	ml	−17.5
GIN AND TONIC	Alcohol	225	ml	−11.0
GIN RICKEY	Alcohol	150	ml	−15.5
GINGER	Condiment	1	tsp	0.5
GINGER SNAPS	Sugar	6	pc	−1.0
GINGERBREAD	Grain	1	pc	0.0
GOAT	Meat/Fish/Poultry	75	g	0.5
GOOSE, Meat and Skin, Baked	Meat/Fish/Poultry	75	g	0.0
GRANOLA BAR,				
Chewy Choc Chip, Quaker	Grain	1	pc	0.5
Oats 'n Honey	Grain	1	pc	−2.0
GRAPEFRUIT, Fresh	Fruit	0.5	pc	13.0
GRAPES, Raw	Fruit	20	pc	4.5
GRAVY	Fat/Oil	50	ml	−2.5
GRAVY MIX, Chicken, Prepared	Fat/Oil	50	ml	0.0
Chicken, made w/Milk/Btr	Fat/Oil	50	ml	−2.5
Mushroom, Prepared	Fat/Oil	50	ml	−0.5
Turkey, made w/Milk & Butter	Fat/Oil	50	ml	−2.5
Turkey, Prepared	Fat/Oil	50	ml	−0.5
GRAVY, Beef, Canned	Fat/Oil	50	ml	1.0
Mix, Pork, Prepared	Fat/Oil	50	ml	−2.0
GREEN PEPPER, Raw	Vegetable	2	pc	37.5
Stuffed with Meat	Meat/Fish/Poultry	1	pc	2.5
GROUPER, Baked	Meat/Fish/Poultry	150	g	3.0
GUACAMOLE	Fruit	50	g	4.5
GUAVA	Fruit	1	pc	21.0
GUM, Bubble	Sugar	5	pc	−6.0
Doublemint, Wrigley's	Sugar	10	pc	−4.5
GUMS, Fruit, Rowntree's	Sugar	10	pc	−3.0
HADDOCK, Baked	Meat/Fish/Poultry	100	g	2.5
Baked Fillet	Meat/Fish/Poultry	150	g	5.0
Floured/Breaded, Fried	Meat/Fish/Poultry	75	g	−1.0

Name	Group	Serving Size		Points
Smoked	Meat/Fish/Poultry	175	g	2.0
HADDOCK FILLETS,				
Frozen, Tesco's	Meat/Fish/Poultry	175	g	6.0
HALIBUT FILLET, Batter-Fried	Meat/Fish/Poultry	75	g	3.5
Baked	Meat/Fish/Poultry	100	g	7.5
Smoked	Meat/Fish/Poultry	75	g	−1.5
HALVAH, Plain	Sugar	25	g	−2.0
HAM, Canned	Meat/Fish/Poultry	100	g	1.0
Canned, Cooked, Ye Olde Oak	Meat/Fish/Poultry	125	g	4.5
HAM SALAD	Meat/Fish/Poultry	125	g	1.0
HAMBURGER PATTY, Grilled	Meat/Fish/Poultry	75	g	0.0
Lean, Fried	Meat/Fish/Poultry	75	g	1.5
Lean, Grilled	Meat/Fish/Poultry	75	g	3.0
HASH	Meat/Fish/Poultry	100	g	−0.5
HAZELNUTS,				
Oil Roasted, Salted	Pulse/Nut/Seed	25	g	0.5
HERRING, Canned	Meat/Fish/Poultry	100	g	1.5
Grilled (Off Bone)	Meat/Fish/Poultry	100	g	3.0
Pickled	Meat/Fish/Poultry	2	pc	0.5
HONEY	Sugar	2	T	−5.5
HORSERADISH	Condiment	1	T	0.0
ICE CREAM, Butter Pecan	Milk/Dairy	125	g	−5.0
Chocolate	Milk/Dairy	60	g	−4.0
Coffee	Milk/Dairy	50	g	−3.5
Dairy, Vanilla	Milk/Dairy	50	g	−2.5
Non Dairy, Neapolitan	Milk/Dairy	60	g	−1.0
Non Dairy, Vanilla, Soft Scoop	Milk/Dairy	60	g	−1.0
Vanilla, Loseley's	Milk/Dairy	75	g	1.0
ICE CREAM SODA	Milk/Dairy	150	ml	−3.5
JAM, Low Cal, All Flavours	Sugar	4	T	−1.0
Robertson's, All Flavours	Fruit	1	T	−5.0
Strawberry	Fruit	2	T	−5.0

Name	Group	Serving Size		Points
JELLY, Cranberry	Fruit	2	T	−5.5
JELLY BEANS	Sugar	15	pc	−5.5
JELLY CUBES, Rowntree's	Fruit	50	g	−5.5
JUICE, Apple	Fruit	150	ml	2.5
Carrot	Vegetable	150	ml	15.0
Grape, Unsweetened	Fruit	150	ml	5.5
Grapefruit, Sweetened, Canned	Fruit	150	ml	7.0
Grapefruit, Unsweetened	Fruit	150	ml	11.0
Lemon	Condiment	1	T	1.0
Lime	Condiment	1	T	0.5
Orange, Fresh Squeezed	Fruit	150	ml	11.5
Orange, Frozen, Reconstituted	Fruit	150	ml	11.0
Tomato	Vegetable	150	ml	24.5
V-8 Vegetable	Vegetable	150	ml	24.5
KALE, Chopped, Cooked	Vegetable	125	g	38.5
KEDGEREE (With Smoked Fish, Rice & Egg)	Meat/Fish/Poultry	100	g	−2.0
KELP	Vegetable	50	g	18.0
KENTUCKY FRIED CHICKEN	Meat/Fish/Poultry	1	pc	−1.0
KENTUCKY FRIED CHICKEN, Mashed Potatoes	Vegetable	100	g	−2.5
KETCHUP, Heinz	Vegetable	2	T	−1.5
KIT KAT BAR, Rowntree's	Sugar	1	pc	−2.0
KIWI FRUIT	Fruit	1	pc	17.0
KOHLRABI, Raw	Vegetable	150	g	24.5
KUMQUAT	Fruit	6	pc	10.0
LAMB, in Hot Onion and Tomato Sauce, Sainsbury's	Meat/Fish/Poultry	100	g	−3.0
LAMB, Neck Fillet, Lean Only	Meat/Fish/Poultry	100	g	0.0
Roast Shoulder, Lean Only	Meat/Fish/Poultry	100	g	−0.5
LAMB CHOP, Loin, Med. Fat, Baked	Meat/Fish/Poultry	50	g	−0.5

Name	Group	Serving Size		Points
LAMB ROAST, Leg, Baked	Meat/Fish/Poultry	75	g	3.5
Leg, Med. Fat, Baked	Meat/Fish/Poultry	75	g	0.5
LAMB SHOULDER, Lean, Baked	Meat/Fish/Poultry	75	g	3.0
Med. Fat, Baked	Meat/Fish/Poultry	75	g	−1.0
LAMB'S KIDNEY, Fried	Meat/Fish/Poultry	100	g	−3.5
LAMB'S LIVER, Fried	Meat/Fish/Poultry	75	g	7.0
LARD	Fat/Oil	1	T	−5.0
LASAGNE, Cooked	Grain	125	g	2.5
Italian Cheese, Fz, Wt Wtchr's	Grain	0.5	pc	1.0
LEEKS, Cooked	Vegetable	100	g	7.5
Raw	Vegetable	2	pc	16.0
LEMON	Condiment	0.25	pc	2.5
LEMONADE, Low Calorie,				
Sainsbury's	Miscellaneous	225	ml	1.0
LENTILS, Split, Boiled	Pulse/Nut/Seed	150	g	8.0
LETTUCE,				
Butterhead/Boston/Bibb,				
Chopped	Vegetable	100	g	34.0
Iceberg	Vegetable	10	pc	18.0
LETTUCE AND TOMATO	Vegetable	125	g	18.5
LIME	Condiment	0.25	pc	1.0
LINGUINE, Buitoni	Grain	60	g	3.0
Spinach High-Protein, Buitoni	Grain	125	g	3.5
LITCHI, Fresh	Fruit	6	pc	16.0
LIVERWURST	Meat/Fish/Poultry	50	g	4.5
LOBSTER, Baked/Grilled with				
Butter	Meat/Fish/Poultry	100	g	−1.0
Floured/Breaded, Fried	Meat/Fish/Poultry	75	g	−0.5
Steamed/Boiled	Meat/Fish/Poultry	175	g	2.5
LUNCHEON MEAT,				
Pork, Prince's	Meat/Fish/Poultry	50	g	−3.0
Turkey Ham	Meat/Fish/Poultry	100	g	2.0

Name	Group	Serving Size		Points
MACADAMIA NUT KERNELS	Pulse/Nut/Seed	8	pc	0.5
MACARONI, Cooked, No Salt	Grain	75	g	3.5
Dry	Grain	25	g	3.5
MACARONI CHEESE	Grain	50	g	0.0
Canned	Milk/Dairy	100	g	1.5
MACKEREL, Baked	Meat/Fish/Poultry	75	g	4.0
MAI TAI	Alcohol	50	ml	−11.5
MALTED MILK POWDER	Milk/Dairy	1	T	1.0
MANDARIN ORANGES,				
Canned, Unsweetened	Fruit	125	g	15.5
MANGO	Fruit	0.5	pc	17.5
MANHATTAN	Alcohol	75	ml	−13.5
MARGARINE	Fat/Oil	15	g	−3.0
Corn Oil	Fat/Oil	15	g	−2.5
Echo	Fat/Oil	15	g	−7.0
Hard	Fat/Oil	15	g	−2.5
Luxury Soft, Sainsbury's	Fat/Oil	15	g	−3.5
Soft, Sainsbury's	Fat/Oil	15	g	−2.5
Soya, Sainsbury's	Fat/Oil	15	g	−3.0
Stork Special Blend	Fat/Oil	15	g	−6.5
Sunflower, Blue Band	Fat/Oil	15	g	−2.5
Sunflower, Flora	Fat/Oil	15	g	−2.5
MARGARITA	Alcohol	75	ml	−13.5
MARJORAM	Condiment	1	tsp	0.5
MARMALADE	Sugar	2	T	−5.0
MARS BAR	Sugar	0.5	pc	−3.5
MARS TWIX	Sugar	2	pc	−4.0
MARSHMALLOWS	Sugar	4	pc	−5.5
MARTINI	Alcohol	75	ml	−15.5
MAYONNAISE	Fat/Oil	1	T	−2.5
Average	Fat/Oil	1	T	−3.5
Homemade with Olive Oil	Fat/Oil	1	T	−3.5

Name	Group	Serving Size		Points
Light Reduced Cal, Hellman's	Fat/Oil	2	T	−3.0
Light Reduced Calorie, Kraft	Fat/Oil	2	T	−2.5
Low Cal	Fat/Oil	2	T	−2.5
Real, Hellman's	Fat/Oil	1	T	−3.5
McDONALD'S				
Chocolate Milk Shake	Milk/Dairy	0.5	pc	−3.0
Hashbrown Potatoes	Vegetable	0.5	pc	−2.0
Regular French Fries	Vegetable	0.25	pc	−0.5
Scrambled Eggs	Milk/Dairy	1	pc	−19.5
Strawberry Milk Shake	Milk/Dairy	0.5	pc	−3.0
Vanilla Milk Shake	Milk/Dairy	0.5	pc	−3.0
MEATBALLS	Meat/Fish/Poultry	2	pc	−0.5
MEATLOAF	Meat/Fish/Poultry	75	g	−0.5
MELON, Cantaloupe	Fruit	0.25	pc	29.0
Honeydew	Fruit	0.25	pc	14.0
MILK,				
Canned, Evaporated, Unsweetened	Milk/Dairy	125	g	1.0
Chocolate	Milk/Dairy	125	g	−0.5
Chocolate, Low Fat (2%)	Milk/Dairy	150	ml	2.5
Evaporated Skimmed, Carnation	Milk/Dairy	150	ml	9.0
Evaporated, Carnation	Milk/Dairy	125	g	1.0
Fresh Channel Island	Milk/Dairy	225	ml	0.5
Goat's	Milk/Dairy	225	ml	1.5
Instant Natural Malted, Carnation	Milk/Dairy	100	ml	−0.5
Non-Dairy, Soy	Pulse/Nut/Seed	225	g	0.5
Semi-skimmed, Fortified	Milk/Dairy	225	ml	6.0
Semi-skimmed, Fresh Pasteurized	Milk/Dairy	225	ml	7.0
Skimmed, Calcium Fortified, Calcia	Milk/Dairy	225	ml	14.0

Name	Group	Serving Size		Points
Skimmed, Calcium Fortified, Vital	Milk/Dairy	225	ml	20.0
Skimmed, Dried, Marvel	Milk/Dairy	40	g	10.0
Skimmed, Fortified, Vitapint	Milk/Dairy	225	ml	10.5
Skimmed, Fresh Pasteurized	Milk/Dairy	225	ml	10.5
Skimmed, Powder, Fort. w/Vitamins	Milk/Dairy	25	g	16.5
Sweetened Condensed, Carnation	Milk/Dairy	75	g	−2.0
Whole, Condensed Sweet, Nestlé	Milk/Dairy	50	g	1.0
Whole, Fresh Pasteurized	Milk/Dairy	225	ml	1.5
Whole, UHT	Milk/Dairy	225	ml	1.0
MILK CHOC BAR, With Almonds	Sugar	1	pc	−3.5
MILK SHAKE,				
w/Skimmed Milk, Nesquik	Milk/Dairy	150	ml	3.5
w/Whole Milk, Nesquik	Milk/Dairy	100	ml	−0.5
MILKY WAY	Sugar	0.5	pc	−4.0
MINT JULEP	Alcohol	50	ml	−15.0
MIXED NUTS,				
Dry Roast, Unsalted	Pulse/Nut/Seed	25	g	1.0
Oil Roasted, Salted	Pulse/Nut/Seed	25	g	1.0
MOLASSES	Sugar	2	T	−3.0
MOUSSE, Chocolate	Sugar	50	g	−5.5
Fruit Flavoured	Milk/Dairy	100	g	0.0
MUFFIN, Bran	Grain	1	pc	3.0
English	Grain	1	pc	4.0
English, with Raisins	Grain	1	pc	4.5
Whole Wheat	Grain	1	pc	6.0
MUSHROOMS, Canned	Vegetable	275	g	13.0
Cooked	Vegetable	100	g	19.0
Fresh	Vegetable	75	g	32.5
Fried w/Breadcrumbs	Vegetable	25	g	−1.0

Name	Group	Serving Size		Points
MUSSELS, Cooked	Meat/Fish/Poultry	175	g	2.0
MUSTARD	Condiment	1	tsp	0.0
MUSTARD POWDER	Condiment	1	tsp	0.5
NACHOS, Cheese/Hot Peppers	Grain	5	pc	1.0
NECTARINE, Fresh	Fruit	1	pc	10.0
NOODLES, Egg, Whole Wheat,				
Uncooked	Grain	25	g	2.0
Spinach, Cooked	Grain	75	g	3.5
NUTMEG	Condiment	1	tsp	0.0
NUTS,				
Mixed, w/Peanuts, Planter's	Pulse/Nut/Seed	25	g	−1.5
OCEAN PERCH, Baked	Meat/Fish/Poultry	100	g	4.5
OCTOPUS, Fried	Meat/Fish/Poultry	75	g	2.0
OIL, Almond	Fat/Oil	1	T	−2.5
Blended Vegetable, Sainsbury's	Fat/Oil	1	T	−2.5
Blended Vegetable, Spry				
Crisp 'n' Dry	Fat/Oil	1	T	−2.5
Cocoa Butter	Fat/Oil	1	T	−5.5
Coconut	Fat/Oil	1	T	−7.0
Corn, Mazola	Fat/Oil	1	T	−3.0
Cottonseed	Fat/Oil	1	T	−3.5
Grapeseed, Sainsbury's	Fat/Oil	1	T	−2.5
Hazelnut	Fat/Oil	1	T	−2.5
Hazelnut, Sainsbury's	Fat/Oil	1	T	−3.0
Linseed	Fat/Oil	1	T	−2.5
Olive	Fat/Oil	1	T	−3.0
Olive, Bertolli	Fat/Oil	1	T	−3.0
Olive, Sainsbury's	Fat/Oil	1	T	−3.0
Palm	Fat/Oil	1	T	−5.0
Palm Kernel	Fat/Oil	1	T	−6.5
Peanut	Fat/Oil	1	T	−3.0
Rapeseed, Sainsbury's	Fat/Oil	1	T	−2.5
Safflower	Fat/Oil	1	T	−2.5

Name	Group	Serving Size		Points
Sesame	Fat/Oil	1	T	−3.0
Sesame Seed, Dufrais	Fat/Oil	1	T	−3.0
Solid Vegetable, Spry Crisp 'n' Dry	Fat/Oil	15	g	−4.0
Soya, Sainsbury's	Fat/Oil	1	T	−3.0
Soybean	Fat/Oil	1	T	−3.0
Sunflower	Fat/Oil	1	T	−2.5
Sunflower, Flora	Fat/Oil	1	T	−2.5
Vegetable, Puritan	Fat/Oil	1	T	−2.5
Walnut	Fat/Oil	1	T	−2.5
Walnut, Sainsbury's	Fat/Oil	1	T	−2.5
Wheat Germ	Fat/Oil	1	T	−3.0
OKRA, Cooked	Vegetable	100	g	31.0
Raw	Vegetable	100	g	26.0
OLD FASHIONED	Alcohol	50	ml	−15.5
OLIVES, Black	Fruit	8	pc	−2.0
Green	Fruit	8	pc	−4.0
Green, in Brine	Fruit	8	pc	−4.5
OMELETTE, Spanish	Milk/Dairy	100	g	−1.5
ONION, Raw	Vegetable	75	g	8.5
Spring	Condiment	2	pc	1.0
ONION POWDER	Condiment	1	tsp	0.5
ONION RINGS, Fried	Vegetable	2	pc	−0.5
ORANGE, Fresh	Fruit	1	pc	13.5
ORANGE MARMALADE, Chiver's	Fruit	1	T	−4.5
OREGANO	Condiment	1	tsp	1.0
OYSTER STEW	Meat/Fish/Poultry	250	g	3.0
OYSTERS, Eastern, Raw	Meat/Fish/Poultry	12	pc	13.0
Fried	Meat/Fish/Poultry	3	pc	1.5
Grilled with Butter	Meat/Fish/Poultry	75	g	7.0
Pacific, Raw	Meat/Fish/Poultry	4	pc	8.0

Name	Group	Serving Size		Points
PANCAKE, Buckwheat	Grain	1	pc	1.0
Plain	Grain	1	pc	0.5
With Fruit	Grain	1	pc	0.5
Whole Wheat	Grain	1	pc	0.5
PAPAYA	Fruit	0.5	pc	20.5
PAPRIKA	Condiment	1	tsp	2.5
PARSLEY, Dried	Condiment	1	tsp	0.5
Fresh	Vegetable	50	g	54.5
PARSNIPS, Cooked	Vegetable	75	g	8.5
Raw	Vegetable	100	g	11.5
PASTA SALAD	Grain	125	g	0.5
PASTRAMI, Beef	Meat/Fish/Poultry	50	g	−2.5
PATÉ, Chicken Liver, Canned	Meat/Fish/Poultry	50	g	0.5
De Foie Gras, Canned (Goose Liver)	Meat/Fish/Poultry	25	g	−1.0
PEACH, Fresh	Fruit	1	pc	11.0
PEACHES, Canned in Juice	Fruit	1	pc	6.5
Canned, Heavy Syrup	Fruit	125	g	0.0
Canned, Unsweetened	Fruit	100	g	10.5
PEANUT BUTTER	Pulse/Nut/Seed	1	T	0.5
Crunchy	Pulse/Nut/Seed	1	T	0.0
Low Sodium	Pulse/Nut/Seed	1	T	1.0
Unsalted	Pulse/Nut/Seed	1	T	1.0
PEANUTS, Chocolate Covered	Pulse/Nut/Seed	25	g	−1.0
Cocktail, Planter's	Pulse/Nut/Seed	25	g	1.0
Dry Roasted, Salted, Planter's	Pulse/Nut/Seed	25	g	1.0
Dry Roasted, Unsalt., Planter's	Pulse/Nut/Seed	25	g	1.5
Oil Roasted, Salted	Pulse/Nut/Seed	25	pc	1.0
Oil Roasted, Unsalted	Pulse/Nut/Seed	25	pc	1.5
Yogurt-covered	Pulse/Nut/Seed	25	g	−1.0
PEAR, Fresh	Fruit	1	pc	4.5
PEARS, Canned, No Sugar	Fruit	125	g	3.5

Name	Group	Serving Size		Points
Canned, Heavy Syrup	Fruit	150	g	−1.0
Dried	Fruit	2	pc	3.0
PEAS, Black-Eyed, Canned	Pulse/Nut/Seed	175	g	9.0
Black-Eyed, Cooked	Pulse/Nut/Seed	175	g	8.5
Canned	Pulse/Nut/Seed	175	g	7.5
Frozen, Cooked	Pulse/Nut/Seed	150	g	14.0
Green, Frozen, Bird's Eye	Pulse/Nut/Seed	200	g	12.0
Processed, Canned, Tesco's	Pulse/Nut/Seed	175	g	8.0
Split, Boiled	Pulse/Nut/Seed	100	g	8.0
Sweet, Canned, Green Giant	Pulse/Nut/Seed	125	g	6.5
PEAS AND CARROTS, Canned	Vegetable	75	g	25.0
Frozen, Cooked	Vegetable	75	g	28.0
PECAN KERNELS	Pulse/Nut/Seed	15	pc	0.0
PECANS, Oil Roasted, Salted	Pulse/Nut/Seed	25	g	−0.5
PEPPER, Black	Condiment	1	tsp	0.5
Cayenne/Red	Condiment	1	tsp	1.5
PEPPERONI	Meat/Fish/Poultry	25	g	−5.0
PEPPERS, Green, Hot Chilli	Condiment	1	T	2.5
Sweet, Red, Raw	Vegetable	2	pc	42.5
PERCH, Fried with Breadcrumbs	Meat/Fish/Poultry	75	g	1.0
PERCH FILLET, Grilled/Baked	Meat/Fish/Poultry	100	g	4.0
PERRIER MINERAL WATER	Miscellaneous	225	ml	0.0
PERSIMMON	Fruit	1	pc	7.5
PHEASANT, without Skin	Meat/Fish/Poultry	100	g	5.5
PICCALILLI	Condiment	1	T	0.0
PICKLE, Sweet, Heinz	Vegetable	1	T	0.5
PIE, Apple	Fruit	0.25	pc	−2.0
Blackberry	Fruit	0.5	pc	−1.5
Blueberry	Fruit	0.5	pc	−2.0
Cherry	Fruit	0.5	pc	−5.0
Custard	Milk/Dairy	0.5	pc	−3.5
Fruit, with Pastry Top and Bottom	Fruit	0.25	pc	−2.0

Name	Group	Serving Size		Points
Lemon Meringue	Fruit	0.25	pc	−4.0
Mince	Fruit	0.25	pc	−1.0
Peach	Fruit	0.5	pc	−2.0
Pecan	Pulse/Nut/Seed	0.5	pc	−3.5
Raspberry	Fruit	0.5	pc	−1.0
Rhubarb, Homemade	Vegetable	0.25	pc	−2.5
Strawberry	Fruit	0.5	pc	−1.5
PIE CRUST	Grain	1	pc	−3.0
PIE FILLING, Apple	Fruit	100	g	−3.0
PIKE, Baked	Meat/Fish/Poultry	175	g	7.5
PINA COLADA	Alcohol	75	ml	−7.5
PINE NUTS, Pignolia	Pulse/Nut/Seed	25	g	1.0
PINEAPPLE,				
Canned, Heavy Syrup	Fruit	125	g	1.0
Fresh	Fruit	75	g	8.0
PISTACHIOS,				
Dry Roasted, Salted	Pulse/Nut/Seed	15	g	0.0
Raw	Pulse/Nut/Seed	25	g	1.0
PIZZA, Cheese & Tomato,				
Homemade	Grain	60	g	0.5
Cheese, Deluxe, Frozen	Grain	1	pc	1.0
Large 16" Ham	Grain	0.5	pc	1.0
Large 16" Veggie	Grain	0.5	pc	1.0
Thick Crust, Frozen	Grain	1	pc	0.5
With Sausage	Grain	0.5	pc	−1.0
PIZZA HUT PEPPERONI PAN				
PIZZA	Grain	0.5	pc	3.0
PLAICE, Baked	Meat/Fish/Poultry	75	g	3.5
PLAICE FILLET, Baked	Meat/Fish/Poultry	125	g	5.5
Baked, Gateway	Meat/Fish/Poultry	100	g	3.0
Breaded, Fried	Meat/Fish/Poultry	75	g	−0.5
PLANTAIN, Cooked	Fruit	75	g	5.5
Fresh	Fruit	0.5	pc	6.0

Name	Group	Serving Size		Points
PLUMS, Fresh	Fruit	2	pc	6.0
Canned, Heavy Syrup	Fruit	150	g	0.0
Canned, Unsweetened	Fruit	125	g	14.0
POMEGRANATE	Fruit	1	pc	3.5
POPCORN, Cooked with Oil	Grain	25	g	0.0
POPPY SEED	Condiment	1	tsp	0.5
PORK, Loin Chop, Grilled, Lean				
and Fat	Meat/Fish/Poultry	75	g	−1.0
Sweet and Sour	Meat/Fish/Poultry	100	g	0.0
PORK CHIPOLATAS, Tesco's	Meat/Fish/Poultry	50	g	−2.0
PORK CHOP, Grilled	Meat/Fish/Poultry	50	g	−0.5
Loin, Lean, Baked	Meat/Fish/Poultry	75	g	3.0
Pan-Fried	Meat/Fish/Poultry	1	pc	−1.0
PORK ROAST, Baked	Meat/Fish/Poultry	50	g	0.0
PORK SPARERIBS	Meat/Fish/Poultry	3	pc	−1.5
PORT	Alcohol	75	ml	−12.5
POTATO, Baked	Vegetable	0.5	pc	8.5
Instant Powder, Made Up	Vegetable	50	g	2.0
POTATO POWDER, Instant,				
Tesco's	Vegetable	25	g	5.5
POTATO SALAD, Home Recipe	Vegetable	75	g	−1.0
POTATOES, Au Gratin	Vegetable	50	g	2.5
Canned	Vegetable	100	g	9.0
Mashed, Home Recipe	Vegetable	50	g	1.0
Scalloped	Vegetable	50	g	2.0
POUSSIN, Roast Meat Only	Meat/Fish/Poultry	100	g	0.5
PRAWNS, Cooked	Meat/Fish/Poultry	15	pc	0.5
PROTEIN POWDER	Miscellaneous	1	T	2.0
PRUNES, Canned, Heavy Syrup	Fruit	50	g	4.5
Cooked, Unsweetened	Fruit	100	g	6.5
Cooked, with Sugar	Fruit	50	g	4.0
Dried	Fruit	4	pc	6.0

Name	Group	Serving Size		Points
PUDDING, Creamed Rice,				
Ambrosia	Milk/Dairy	200	g	1.0
Milk	Grain	100	g	0.5
Tapioca	Milk/Dairy	80	g	−0.5
QUAIL, without Skin	Meat/Fish/Poultry	100	g	6.0
QUICHE, Cheese	Milk/Dairy	0.5	pc	−6.0
Cheese and Egg	Milk/Dairy	50	g	−2.5
Cheese & Egg w/Wholemeal				
Pastry	Milk/Dairy	50	g	−2.5
Cheese/Bacon	Milk/Dairy	0.25	pc	−4.5
Lorraine	Milk/Dairy	50	g	−2.5
QUINCE	Fruit	1	pc	6.0
RABBIT,				
Domestic, Breaded, Fried	Meat/Fish/Poultry	75	g	3.0
Stewed	Meat/Fish/Poultry	75	g	2.0
Wild	Meat/Fish/Poultry	75	g	3.0
RADISHES, Raw	Vegetable	100	g	29.0
RAISINS	Fruit	35	g	4.0
Carob-covered	Fruit	25	g	−1.0
Chocolate-covered	Fruit	25	g	−1.5
Thompson Seedless	Fruit	2	T	3.0
RASPBERRIES, Fresh	Fruit	75	g	12.5
RAVIOLI, Canned in Tomato				
Sauce	Grain	150	g	1.5
RED SNAPPER, Baked	Meat/Fish/Poultry	175	g	7.0
RHUBARB, Cooked, with Sugar	Vegetable	75	g	−2.5
RICE, Brown, Cooked w/o Salt	Grain	100	g	4.0
Pilaf	Grain	100	g	2.0
Spanish	Grain	125	g	4.0
White, Cooked, w/o Salt	Grain	100	g	3.0
White, w/Added Salt	Grain	100	g	3.0
ROLL, Cracked Wheat	Grain	1	pc	3.0

Name	Group	Serving Size		Points
French, Part Cooked	Grain	0.5	pc	2.5
Rye	Grain	1	pc	3.5
Starch Reduced	Grain	30	g	2.0
White	Grain	1	pc	2.0
Wholemeal	Grain	1	pc	4.5
ROSEMARY	Condiment	1	tsp	0.5
RUM	Alcohol	75	ml	−16.5
RUM AND CARBONATED				
BEVERAGE	Alcohol	75	ml	−10.5
RUM, Hot Buttered	Alcohol	75	ml	−12.5
RUNNER BEANS, Boiled	Vegetable	125	g	24.5
SAGE	Condiment	1	tsp	0.5
SALAD, Spinach, w/Egg/Bacon/				
Tomato	Vegetable	75	g	4.0
Three Bean	Pulse/Nut/Seed	125	g	1.5
Tossed, No Dressing	Vegetable	125	g	33.0
Tossed, with Tomato	Vegetable	125	g	21.5
Waldorf	Fruit	125	g	−2.0
SALAD CREAM,				
Average, Reduced Calorie	Fat/Oil	4	T	−2.5
SALAMI, Beef	Meat/Fish/Poultry	50	g	0.0
Black Peppered, Tesco's	Meat/Fish/Poultry	50	g	−3.5
Pork	Meat/Fish/Poultry	4	pc	1.0
SALMON, Baked with Butter	Meat/Fish/Poultry	75	g	2.0
Baked/Grilled	Meat/Fish/Poultry	75	g	5.5
Canned in Water	Meat/Fish/Poultry	100	g	6.5
Scotch Smoked	Meat/Fish/Poultry	100	g	0.5
Smoked	Meat/Fish/Poultry	75	g	3.0
Steamed/Poached	Meat/Fish/Poultry	75	g	7.5
SALMON AND SHRIMP PASTE,				
Tesco's	Meat/Fish/Poultry	25	g	1.5
SALMON TROUT,				
Scotch Smoked	Meat/Fish/Poultry	100	g	0.0

Name	Group	Serving Size		Points
SALT	Condiment	1	tsp	0.0
SALT, Lo	Condiment	1	tsp	0.0
SALT PORK, Raw	Meat/Fish/Poultry	25	g	−4.0
SAMOSA, Meat-Filled	Meat/Fish/Poultry	50	g	−2.5
SANDWICH, BLT, White Bread	Meat/Fish/Poultry	0.5	pc	1.0
BLT, Whole Wheat Bread	Meat/Fish/Poultry	0.5	pc	2.0
Chicken Salad, White Bread	Meat/Fish/Poultry	0.5	pc	3.5
Chicken Salad, Whole Wheat	Meat/Fish/Poultry	0.5	pc	4.0
Chicken, White Bread	Meat/Fish/Poultry	0.5	pc	2.0
Chicken, Whole Wheat Bread	Meat/Fish/Poultry	0.5	pc	2.0
Corned Beef, Rye Bread	Meat/Fish/Poultry	0.5	pc	1.5
Egg Salad, White Bread	Milk/Dairy	0.5	pc	−3.5
Egg Salad, Whole Wheat Bread	Milk/Dairy	0.5	pc	−3.0
Grilled Cheese, White	Milk/Dairy	0.5	pc	0.0
Ham Salad, White	Meat/Fish/Poultry	0.5	pc	−0.5
Ham Salad, Whole Wheat	Meat/Fish/Poultry	0.5	pc	0.0
Ham/Cheese, Rye	Meat/Fish/Poultry	0.5	pc	0.5
Ham/Cheese, White	Meat/Fish/Poultry	0.5	pc	0.0
Ham/Cheese, Whole Wheat	Meat/Fish/Poultry	0.5	pc	0.5
Peanut Butter, White	Pulse/Nut/Seed	0.5	pc	1.5
Peanut Butter, Whole Wheat	Pulse/Nut/Seed	0.5	pc	2.0
Peanut Butter/Jelly, White	Pulse/Nut/Seed	0.5	pc	0.5
Peanut Butter/Jelly, Whole Wheat	Pulse/Nut/Seed	0.5	pc	0.5
Roast Beef, Hot	Meat/Fish/Poultry	0.5	pc	1.0
Tuna Salad, White	Meat/Fish/Poultry	0.5	pc	3.0
Tuna Salad, Whole Wheat	Meat/Fish/Poultry	0.5	pc	3.5
Turkey, White Bread	Meat/Fish/Poultry	0.5	pc	1.5
Turkey, Whole Wheat Bread	Meat/Fish/Poultry	0.5	pc	2.5
SARDINE AND TOMATO PASTE, Tesco's	Meat/Fish/Poultry	25	g	1.5
SARDINES, Canned in Oil	Meat/Fish/Poultry	3	pc	4.5
Canned, Tomato Sauce	Meat/Fish/Poultry	6	pc	3.5

Name	Group	Serving Size		Points
SAUCE MIX, Bearnaise,				
w/Milk-Butter	Fat/Oil	75	g	−5.5
Curry, w/Milk	Fat/Oil	75	g	0.0
Mushroom, Made w/Milk	Fat/Oil	75	g	1.0
Stroganoff, w/Milk & Water	Fat/Oil	75	g	1.5
Sweet and Sour, Prepared	Fat/Oil	75	g	0.0
SAUCE, Barbeque	Condiment	1	T	0.0
Bread, Homemade with Skim				
Milk	Fat/Oil	2	T	3.0
Butterscotch	Sugar	2	T	−4.5
Cheese	Milk/Dairy	4	T	−5.5
Cheese, Packet Mix made				
w/Skim Milk	Fat/Oil	100	ml	0.5
Chilli	Condiment	1	T	1.0
Chocolate	Sugar	2	T	−5.0
Chocolate Fudge	Sugar	2	T	−3.5
Hollandaise	Fat/Oil	4	T	−5.0
Soy	Condiment	1	tsp	0.0
Spaghetti, Meatless	Vegetable	150	g	4.0
Sweet and Sour	Condiment	1	T	−1.5
Tartare	Fat/Oil	2	T	−3.5
Tartare, Kraft	Fat/Oil	1	T	−0.5
Tomato, Canned	Vegetable	125	g	17.5
White	Fat/Oil	50	ml	−1.0
White, Packet Mix made				
w/Skim Milk	Fat/Oil	125	ml	4.5
Worcestershire	Condiment	1	tsp	1.0
SAUERKRAUT, Canned	Vegetable	250	g	17.0
SAUSAGE, Italian	Meat/Fish/Poultry	50	g	−0.5
Polish	Meat/Fish/Poultry	50	g	0.0
Pork, Wall's Best English	Meat/Fish/Poultry	50	g	−2.5
SCALLOPS, Baked/Grilled	Meat/Fish/Poultry	175	g	4.0
Fried	Meat/Fish/Poultry	75	g	1.0

Name	Group	Serving Size		Points
SCAMPI	Meat/Fish/Poultry	3	pc	−1.0
SCREWDRIVER	Alcohol	225	ml	−9.5
SEEDS, Sesame	Pulse/Nut/Seed	40	g	0.0
Sunflower, Unsalted	Pulse/Nut/Seed	40	g	4.5
SESAME BUTTER (TAHINI)	Pulse/Nut/Seed	25	g	1.5
SHALLOTS, Raw	Vegetable	50	g	8.5
SHARK, Mixed Species, Raw	Meat/Fish/Poultry	100	g	4.0
SHEPHERD'S PIE,				
Frozen, Tesco's	Meat/Fish/Poultry	150	g	0.0
SHERRY, Dry	Alcohol	100	ml	−15.5
Sweet	Alcohol	100	ml	−14.0
SHORTBREAD	Grain	30	g	−2.5
SHORTENING,				
Polyunsaturated, White Flora	Fat/Oil	15	g	−3.0
Vegetable, Trex	Fat/Oil	15	g	−3.5
SINGAPORE SLING	Alcohol	150	ml	−13.5
SKATE WING, Fried in Batter	Meat/Fish/Poultry	150	g	−1.5
SMELT, Rainbow, Baked	Meat/Fish/Poultry	100	g	4.5
SNAILS	Meat/Fish/Poultry	100	g	4.0
SOFT DRINK, 7-Up	Sugar	325	ml	−5.5
Coke	Sugar	325	ml	−6.0
Cream Soda	Sugar	325	ml	−5.5
Ginger Ale	Sugar	325	ml	−5.0
SOLE, Baked	Meat/Fish/Poultry	175	g	6.0
SOLE FILLETS,				
Lemon, Frozen, Sainsbury's	Meat/Fish/Poultry	150	g	3.0
SOUFFLÉ, Cheese	Milk/Dairy	75	g	−3.0
Spinach	Vegetable	75	g	−3.0
SOUP, Bean	Pulse/Nut/Seed	250	g	3.5
Bean, Black	Pulse/Nut/Seed	250	g	5.0
Beef	Meat/Fish/Poultry	250	g	4.0
Beef, Heinz	Meat/Fish/Poultry	250	g	1.0

Name	Group	Serving Size		Points
Beef & Veg, Main Course, Campbell's	Meat/Fish/Poultry	250	g	1.0
Beef Noodle	Meat/Fish/Poultry	250	g	1.0
Chicken	Meat/Fish/Poultry	250	g	1.5
Chicken & Mushroom, Heinz	Meat/Fish/Poultry	250	g	−4.0
Chicken & Veg Main Course, Campbell's	Meat/Fish/Poultry	250	g	−1.0
Chicken Gumbo	Meat/Fish/Poultry	175	g	5.5
Chicken Noodle	Meat/Fish/Poultry	250	g	0.5
Chowder, Fish	Meat/Fish/Poultry	175	g	1.0
Clam Chowder	Meat/Fish/Poultry	250	g	−0.5
Cream of Asparagus	Vegetable	125	g	1.0
Cream of Celery	Vegetable	125	g	−0.5
Cream of Chicken	Meat/Fish/Poultry	250	g	0.0
Cream of Chicken, Spec. Rec., Heinz	Meat/Fish/Poultry	250	g	−3.5
Cream of Mushroom	Vegetable	75	g	−1.0
Cream of Mushroom, Campbell's	Vegetable	100	g	−4.5
Cream of Mushroom, Campbell's, Low Sodium	Vegetable	50	g	−1.0
Cream of Tomato, Canned, Heinz	Vegetable	100	g	−1.0
French Onion	Vegetable	225	g	−3.5
Green Pea, Campbell's	Pulse/Nut/Seed	225	g	2.5
Lentil	Pulse/Nut/Seed	225	g	5.5
Lentil, with Ham	Pulse/Nut/Seed	250	g	4.5
Minestrone	Vegetable	225	g	3.5
Minestrone, Homemade	Pulse/Nut/Seed	200	g	4.0
Onion	Vegetable	250	g	−1.5
Pea	Pulse/Nut/Seed	250	g	4.0
Potato	Vegetable	125	g	0.5

Name	Group	Serving Size		Points
Seafood Gumbo	Meat/Fish/Poultry	450	g	3.5
Tomato	Vegetable	250	g	2.5
Tomato, Campbell's	Vegetable	225	g	0.5
Vegetable	Vegetable	250	g	12.0
Vegetable Beef	Vegetable	250	g	4.5
Vegetable, Campbell's	Vegetable	225	g	2.0
Vegetable, No Salt	Vegetable	225	g	13.0
SOUP MIX, Cream of Mushroom	Vegetable	225	g	−2.5
Tomato, Cup-A-Soup	Vegetable	225	g	−2.5
SOYBEANS, Cooked	Pulse/Nut/Seed	125	g	7.0
Dry	Pulse/Nut/Seed	25	g	7.5
SPAGHETTI, Canned in Tomato				
Sauce	Grain	200	g	−0.5
Cooked	Grain	75	g	3.0
SPAM	Meat/Fish/Poultry	50	g	−1.5
SPINACH, Fresh, Cooked	Vegetable	175	g	53.5
Frozen, Cooked	Vegetable	150	g	42.5
Raw, Chopped	Vegetable	100	g	75.0
Whole Leaf, Fz, Bird's Eye	Vegetable	175	g	57.0
SPONGE CAKE, Chocolate, with				
Icing	Grain	30	g	−3.5
SPREAD, Dairy Master, Golden				
Churn	Fat/Oil	15	g	−4.5
Golden Churn, Kraft	Fat/Oil	15	g	−3.5
Half Fat, Anchor	Fat/Oil	30	g	−6.0
Krona	Fat/Oil	15	g	−5.5
Krona Spreadable	Fat/Oil	15	g	−5.0
Low Fat, Clover Light	Fat/Oil	30	g	−3.5
Low Fat, Delight	Fat/Oil	30	g	−2.5
Low Fat, Gold	Fat/Oil	30	g	−2.5
Low Fat, Unsalted, Gold	Fat/Oil	30	g	−2.5
Mello, Kraft	Fat/Oil	30	g	−2.5

Name	Group	Serving Size		Points
Reduced Fat, Clover	Fat/Oil	15	g	−2.5
Red. Fat, Slightly Salted, Clover	Fat/Oil	15	g	−2.5
Reduced Fat, Stork Light Blend	Fat/Oil	15	g	−6.5
Summer County	Fat/Oil	15	g	−5.5
Sunflower, Low Fat, Flora Ex. Light	Fat/Oil	30	g	−2.0
Sunflower, Red. Fat, Vitalite Light	Fat/Oil	30	g	−2.5
Very Low Fat, Gold Lowest	Fat/Oil	50	g	−1.5
Very Low Fat, Outline	Fat/Oil	50	g	−1.5
Willow	Fat/Oil	15	g	−5.0
SPRING ONIONS	Vegetable	10	pc	24.0
SQUID, Boiled	Meat/Fish/Poultry	175	g	−1.5
Fried	Meat/Fish/Poultry	75	g	0.0
Raw	Meat/Fish/Poultry	175	g	2.0
STINGER	Alcohol	50	ml	−12.5
STOUT	Alcohol	325	ml	−8.5
STRAWBERRIES, Fresh	Fruit	150	g	19.0
Frozen, Unsweetened	Fruit	150	g	17.0
STUFFING	Grain	100	g	−1.5
STURGEON, Steamed	Meat/Fish/Poultry	100	g	5.5
SUET, Shredded Beef, Copperfields	Fat/Oil	15	g	−2.5
SUGAR, Brown	Sugar	2	T	−5.0
Raw	Sugar	2	T	−5.0
White	Sugar	2	T	−6.0
SUSHI/RAW FISH	Meat/Fish/Poultry	175	g	2.5
SWEET POTATO/YAM, Baked	Vegetable	0.5	pc	12.0
SWEETBREADS	Meat/Fish/Poultry	75	g	−52.0
SWISS CHARD, Cooked	Vegetable	175	g	42.0
SWORDFISH FILLET, Breaded, Fried	Meat/Fish/Poultry	75	g	1.0

Name	Group	Serving Size		Points
Baked	Meat/Fish/Poultry	75	g	6.5
SYRUP, Maple	Sugar	2	T	−5.0
TANGERINE	Fruit	1	pc	13.0
TARRAGON	Condiment	1	tsp	0.5
TEA, Decaffeinated	Miscellaneous	225	ml	0.0
Herb	Miscellaneous	150	ml	0.5
Infused	Miscellaneous	225	ml	−3.0
TEQUILA SUNRISE	Alcohol	150	ml	−10.0
THYME	Condiment	1	tsp	0.5
TOFFEE ASSORTMENT,				
Sainsbury's	Sugar	30	g	−5.5
TOFU	Pulse/Nut/Seed	125	g	5.0
TOM COLLINS	Alcohol	225	ml	−14.0
TOMATO, Fresh	Vegetable	1	pc	30.0
TOMATO PURÉE, Canned	Vegetable	4	T	20.0
TOMATOES, Canned,				
Peeled, Drained, Prince's	Vegetable	125	g	40.5
Canned	Vegetable	125	g	23.0
TONIC WATER, Sweetened	Sugar	325	ml	−5.5
TOPPING,				
Dream, Bird's w/Skim Milk	Milk/Dairy	65	g	−2.5
Dream, Bird's w/Whole Milk	Milk/Dairy	50	g	−3.5
Whipped	Milk/Dairy	4	T	−5.5
TORTILLA CHIPS	Grain	15	pc	0.5
TRAIL MIX	Pulse/Nut/Seed	25	g	2.0
TROUT, Baked	Meat/Fish/Poultry	75	g	5.0
TUNA, Canned in Oil	Meat/Fish/Poultry	100	g	2.0
Canned in Water	Meat/Fish/Poultry	150	g	7.5
Fresh, Grilled	Meat/Fish/Poultry	75	g	6.5
TUNA NOODLE CASSEROLE	Meat/Fish/Poultry	200	g	3.5
TUNA SALAD	Meat/Fish/Poultry	100	g	3.0
TURKEY, Dark Meat and Skin,				
Baked	Meat/Fish/Poultry	100	g	1.0

Name	Group	Serving Size		Points
Dark Meat, Baked w/o Skin	Meat/Fish/Poultry	75	g	3.0
Light Meat and Skin, Baked	Meat/Fish/Poultry	100	g	2.5
Light Meat Baked w/o Skin	Meat/Fish/Poultry	75	g	4.5
Light/Dk Meat, w/o Skin, Baked	Meat/Fish/Poultry	75	g	3.5
TURKEY AND HAM PIE, Tiffany's Uppercrust	Meat/Fish/Poultry	100	g	0.5
TURKEY BREAST IN JELLY, Sainsbury's	Meat/Fish/Poultry	175	g	4.0
TURKEY BREAST, Cured, Tesco's	Meat/Fish/Poultry	150	g	7.0
Premium Sliced, Tesco's	Meat/Fish/Poultry	125	g	6.5
TURKEY POT PIE	Meat/Fish/Poultry	0.5	pc	0.5
TURKEY ROLL, Light Meat	Meat/Fish/Poultry	75	g	3.0
TURMERIC	Condiment	1	tsp	0.5
TURNIP TOPS, Boiled	Vegetable	150	g	79.0
TURNIPS, Cooked	Vegetable	150	g	19.5
Raw	Vegetable	75	g	18.0
TURNOVER, Fruit	Grain	1	pc	−1.5
VANILLA EXTRACT	Condiment	1	tsp	0.0
VEAL CHOP, Med. Fat, Fried	Meat/Fish/Poultry	75	g	−0.5
VEAL CUTLET, Med. Fat, Braised	Meat/Fish/Poultry	75	g	1.0
VEAL CUTLET/STEAK, Lean, Braised	Meat/Fish/Poultry	75	g	3.5
VEAL PARMIGIANI	Meat/Fish/Poultry	0.5	pc	−1.5
VEAL ROAST, Lean, Braised	Meat/Fish/Poultry	75	g	2.0
Med. Fat, Braised	Meat/Fish/Poultry	75	g	0.5
VEGEBURGERS	Pulse/Nut/Seed	1	pc	1.5
VEGETABLES, Japan Style, Fz, Bird's Eye	Vegetable	100	g	2.5
Mixed, Canned	Vegetable	75	g	22.0

Name	Group	Serving Size		Points
Mixed, Fz, Bird's Eye	Vegetable	100	g	18.0
Mixed, Fz, Cooked	Vegetable	75	g	18.0
VENISON, Baked	Meat/Fish/Poultry	100	g	8.5
VERMOUTH, Dry	Alcohol	100	ml	−14.0
Sweet	Alcohol	75	ml	−11.5
VINEGAR	Condiment	1	T	0.0
VODKA	Alcohol	50	ml	−16.5
WAFFLES	Grain	1	pc	4.0
WALNUTS	Pulse/Nut/Seed	12	pc	0.5
WATER BISCUITS	Grain	30	g	0.5
WATER CHESTNUTS, Canned	Vegetable	100	g	5.5
WATERCRESS	Vegetable	20	pc	52.5
WATERMELON	Fruit	150	g	10.5
WHEAT GERM	Grain	25	g	10.5
WHISKY	Alcohol	50	ml	−16.5
WHISKY SOUR	Alcohol	75	ml	−19.0
WHITE FISH, In Parsley Sauce, Tesco's	Meat/Fish/Poultry	150	g	4.5
WHITE RUSSIAN	Alcohol	50	ml	−13.0
WHITING, Grilled, Baked	Meat/Fish/Poultry	100	g	2.0
WINE, Red	Alcohol	100	ml	−15.5
White, Dry	Alcohol	100	ml	−14.0
White, Sweet	Alcohol	100	ml	−13.0
WINE SPRITZER	Alcohol	150	ml	−14.5
YEAST, Brewer's	Miscellaneous	1	T	3.5
Dry Active	Miscellaneous	1	pc	0.0
YOGURT, B'Active Set, w/Vits C, A & D, Chambourcy	Milk/Dairy	125	g	4.5
Frozen	Milk/Dairy	100	g	1.5
Greek, Cow's	Milk/Dairy	125	g	0.0
Greek, Sheep, Total	Milk/Dairy	125	g	0.0
Low Fat Set, w/Natural Fruit, Sains.	Milk/Dairy	125	g	2.0

Low Fat, Apricot, Tesco's	Milk/Dairy	150	g	1.5
Low Fat, Blackberry & Apple, Tesco's	Milk/Dairy	150	g	1.5
Low Fat, Blackcurrant, Tesco's	Milk/Dairy	150	g	2.0
Low Fat, Fruits of the Forest, Tesco's	Milk/Dairy	150	g	1.5
Low Fat, Hazelnut, Tesco's	Milk/Dairy	150	g	2.5
Low Fat, Natural, St Ivel	Milk/Dairy	175	g	8.0
Low Fat, Orange, Ski	Milk/Dairy	150	g	2.5
Low Fat, Plain	Milk/Dairy	175	g	8.5
Low Fat, Plain, Eden Vale	Milk/Dairy	150	g	7.0
Low Fat, Plain, Sainsbury's	Milk/Dairy	150	g	8.0
Low Fat, Raspberry, Ski	Milk/Dairy	150	g	2.5
Lowfat, Peach	Milk/Dairy	125	g	−0.5
Natural, Thick Set, Sainsbury's	Milk/Dairy	150	g	3.0
Thick 'n' Creamy, Sainsbury's	Milk/Dairy	125	g	0.0
Very Low Fat, Black Cherry, Shape	Milk/Dairy	225	g	10.0
Very Low Fat, Plain, Shape	Milk/Dairy	200	g	8.5
Very Low Fat, Strawberry, Sains.	Milk/Dairy	250	g	10.0
Very Low Fat, Strawberry, Shape	Milk/Dairy	250	g	10.5
YOGURT DRINK, Strawberry, Yop	Milk/Dairy	100	ml	6.5

POSTSCRIPT

If your life-style does not control your body, eventually your body will control your life-style. The choice is yours.

Ern Baxter
Author of *I Almost Died*

We all pay lip service to the value of good health habits. We hear retired people say things such as, 'As long as you've got your health . . . ,' and we agree, even if we're years from thinking that anything could go wrong with our health. But as the years go by, and we begin to see how things *can* go wrong – how friends and relations can be stricken by chronic illness – we begin to appreciate the notion that good health is a very valuable commodity. Unfortunately, for many people, it can be too late.

Ern Baxter had a heart attack in middle age that frightened him more than he ever thought he could be frightened. Suddenly, he faced the possibility of his life ending much sooner than he'd thought. After a sea change in his attitudes about health and fitness, he rehabilitated himself to the point where he feels better than he had ever felt before his brush with death. I've quoted above from his book because I think his comment crystallizes everything you need to know about respecting your body and doing your best to keep it in optimum condition.

Good nutrition is a major component of a healthy life. I think that Nutripoints will help you achieve the best level of nutrition you've ever experienced. I would like to point out that to achieve an optimum sense of well-being, you must make both exercise and stress control part of your regimen. I strongly suggest that you investigate these areas and adopt some form of exercise, as well as techniques for stress control, so that you can enjoy the maximum benefits of Nutripoints.

Some excellent books on exercise include Dr Kenneth Cooper's *Aerobics* (Bantam, 1968) and *Aerobics Program for Total Well-Being* (M. Evans, 1982); Casey Meyer's *Aerobic Walking* (Vintage, 1987); and Arthur Turock's *Getting Physical* (Doubleday, 1984).

For a good introduction to stress management I recommend Dr Robert Eliot's *Is It Worth Dying For?* (Bantam, 1984); Drs Kriegel and Kriegel's *The C Zone: Peak Performance Under Pressure* (Fawcett, Columbine, 1984); Dr Herbert Benson's *Beyond the Relaxation Response* (Berkeley, 1984); and Alan Lakein's *How to Get Control of Your Time and Your Life* (Signet, New American Library, 1974).

As a final note, I'd like to say that I don't think nutrition, exercise, and stress control are the most important things in life. I think eating should be pleasurable. I think exercise should be fun. I think time spent with loved ones and devoted to spiritual goals are at the core of a happy life. But I've seen that optimum health can affect life for the better, and I know that good health is achievable. So I want to convince you that it's a gift you can give yourself. It can enhance every other aspect of your life. I hope that *Nutripoints* will make your ultimate life goals easier to achieve.

REFERENCES

Association of Vitamin Chemists, The. *Methods of Vitamin Assay*. New York: Interscience Publishers, 1966

Bland, Dr Jeffrey. *Nutraerobics*. San Francisco: Harper & Row, 1983.

Brody, Jane. *Jane Brody's Nutrition Book*. New York: Norton, 1981.

Carper, Jean. *Jean Carper's Total Nutrition Guide*. New York: Bantam, 1987.

Connor, Sonja L., and William Connor. *The New American Diet*. New York: Simon & Schuster, 1986.

Hendler, Sheldon Saul, MD. *The Complete Guide to Anti-Aging Nutrients*. New York: Simon & Schuster, 1984.

Katch, Frank I., and William D. McArdle. *Nutrition, Weight Control, and Exercise*. Boston: Houghton Mifflin, 1988.

Last, John M., MD, Ed. *Maxcy-Rosenau: Public Health and Preventive Medicine*, 11th ed. New York: Appleton-Century-Crofts, 1980.

Mayer, Jean. *A Diet for Living*. New York: David McKay, 1975.

National Research Council. *Diet and Health: Implications for Reducing Chronic Disease*. Washington, DC: National Academy Press, 1989.

National Research Council. *Recommended Dietary Allowances*, 9th revised ed. Washington, DC: National Academy of Sciences, 1980.

Paige, David MD, ed. *Manual of Clinical Nutrition*. Pleasantville, NJ: Nutrition Publications, 1983.

Pennington, Jean A. T., and Helen Nichols-Church. *Food Values of Portions Commonly Used*, 14th ed. New York: Harper & Row, 1985.

Saltman, Paul, Joel Gurin, and Ira Mothner. *California Nutrition Book*. Boston: Little Brown, 1987.

Schmid, Dr Ronald F. *Traditional Foods Are Your Best Medicine*. New York: Ballantine, 1987.

Stunkard, Albert J., MD, ed. *Obesity*. Philadelphia: W. B. Saunders, 1980.

United States Department of Agriculture. *Composition of Foods*, Agricultural Handbooks 8-1 through 8-17 and 8-21. Washington, DC: USDA, 1978–1989.

United States Department of Agriculture. *Nutritive Value of Foods*, Home and Garden Bulletin No. 72, Washington, DC: U.S. Government Printing Office, 1988.

United States Department of Health and Human Services, Public Health Service, Centers For Disease Control. *Foodborne Disease Surveillance*, Annual Summary, 1982. Atlanta: U.S. Department of Health and Human Services, issued September 1985.

Walford, Roy L., MD. *The 120-Year Diet*. New York: Simon & Schuster, 1986.

Weiner, Michael A. *The Way of the Skeptical Nutritionist*. New York: Macmillan, 1981.

Whalen, Dr Elizabeth, and Dr Frederic J. Stare. *The 100% Natural, Purely Organic, Cholesterol-Free, Megavitamin, Low-Carbohydrate Nutrition Hoax*. New York: Atheneum, 1983.